AMERICAN MEDICAL ASSOCIATION
ESSENTIAL GUIDE TO
MENOPAUSE

Each woman's experience with menopause is unique. Identifying the possible symptoms of menopause is complicated by the fact that menopause usually occurs at a time when the body is undergoing changes related to normal aging, such as wrinkles, stiff joints, and brittle bones. By making lifestyle changes and taking good care of yourself, particularly in your middle years, you can slow many of the changes that occur as you grow older. A healthful diet, weight-bearing exercise, and use of hormone replacement therapy can help women stay in good health as they go through menopause and the years beyond it. Vital information on preventing heart disease and osteoporosis is also included in this invaluable guide.

Trust the American Medical Association to bring you current, accessible medical information on all aspects of this life-changing condition in the *American Medical Association Essential Guide to Menopause.*

American
Medical
Association

ESSENTIAL

GUIDE

TO

MENOPAUSE

POCKET BOOKS
New York   London   Toronto   Sydney   Singapore

The information, procedures, and recommendations in this book are not intended as a substitute for the medical advice of a trained health professional. All matters regarding your health require medical supervision. Consult your physician before adopting the suggestions in this book, as well as about any condition that may require diagnosis or medical attention.

In addition, statements made by the author regarding certain products do not constitute an endorsement of any product, service, or organization by the author or publisher, each of whom specifically disclaims any responsibility for any liability, loss, or risk, personal or otherwise, which is incurred as a consequence, directly or indirectly, of the use and application of any of the contents of this book or any of the products mentioned herein.

POCKET BOOKS, a division of Simon & Schuster Inc.
1230 Avenue of the Americas, New York, NY 10020

Copyright © 1998 by American Medical Association

Originally published in trade paperback in 1998 by Pocket Books

All rights reserved, including the right to reproduce this book or portions thereof in any form whatsoever. For information address Pocket Books, 1230 Avenue of the Americas, New York, NY 10020

ISBN: 0-7434-0358-4

First Pocket Books mass market paperback printing April 2000

10 9 8 7 6 5 4 3 2

POCKET and colophon are registered trademarks of Simon & Schuster Inc.

Cover design by Elizabeth Van Itallie
Cover photo by Jim Cummins/FPG International

Printed in the U.S.A.

American Medical Association

Physicians dedicated to the health of America

Foreword

Not too many years ago, menopause was considered almost a taboo topic, and there was little information available about what to expect or how women could help themselves through menopause. Women today are greatly interested in preventive medicine for themselves and their families, and information is now widely available on the experience of menopause and the choices a woman can make.

Menopause is a natural condition of life, in which a woman's menstrual periods stop and other changes occur in her body. Menopause is not a disease or disorder, but certain treatments can help alleviate problem symptoms of menopause and help prevent disorders such as heart disease and osteoporosis. The *American Medical Association Essential Guide to Menopause* offers clear, medically accurate, up-to-date information on treatment options such as hormone replacement therapy. Stress management, weight-bearing exercise, and nutritional changes are also very useful to women going through menopause.

AMA member physicians proudly offer this information to women who want to stay healthy and active and who are proactive about their own health. If you have access to the Internet, look for more information about family health and about doctors on the AMA website at **http://www.ama-assn.org**; if you need a physician, you can access information by the doctor's name or by specialty under Physician Select: Online Doctor Finder.

The American Medical Association wishes you and your family the best of health.

Nancy W. Dickey, MD
President, American Medical Association

The American Medical Association

Acknowledgments

Steven N. Blair, PED, Exercise/Fitness
Linda Bresolin, PhD, American Medical Association
Janis Donnaud, Literary Agent
Sue Finn, PhD, RD, SADA, Nutrition
Irwin M. Siegel, MD, Orthopedics
Ramona Slupik, MD, Gynecology
Julian Ullman, MD, Gynecology
Rolin Graphics, Inc., Minneapolis

Contents

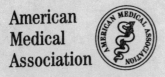

American
Medical
Association

ESSENTIAL
GUIDE
TO
MENOPAUSE

Introduction

Women tend to view menopause with mixed emotions. You may be pleased at the prospect of no more menstrual periods and a sex life free of contraception and the fear of pregnancy, but you may also have some regrets about no longer being able to bear children. You may be focusing on possible unpleasant symptoms or worrying that menopause will inevitably cause health problems such as osteoporosis, heart disease, and cancer. You may think of menopause as the end of life as you know it, or you may see it as an opportunity for a new beginning. Each woman's attitudes and experiences regarding menopause are a little different.

Recent advances in the understanding of the biological effects of menopause, primarily the loss of estrogen, have led to many new treatments that can postpone or reverse some of these effects. Most doctors believe that hormone replacement therapy to replace estrogen that is naturally reduced at menopause is beneficial for most women. Taking estrogen can cut in half a woman's risk of heart disease (the number one killer of women), help keep her bones strong, and may also reduce her risk of Alzheimer's disease.

In addition to new medical treatments for conditions such as osteoporosis, simple lifestyle changes can also help women stay healthy. For example, doing weight-bearing exercises and taking calcium supplements can help lower the rate at which a woman loses bone density (although neither of these measures, alone or in combination, is as effective as estrogen). Along with exercise, eating a low-fat diet that is rich in fruits, vegetables, and whole grains can significantly reduce the risk of heart disease, stroke, and many cancers.

Another significant factor in improving health and quality of life during menopause is a positive outlook. Women who are optimistic and who have a positive approach to life are at less risk for all kinds of medical problems, including depression. A positive attitude will help you to take control of your health and your future.

If you are approaching menopause—or perhaps experiencing hot flashes, fatigue, mood swings, or irregular periods—the *American Medical Association Essential Guide to Menopause* will provide accurate, up-to-date information to help you understand and deal with these changes. A glossary at the back of the book defines many common terms related to menopause and women's health.

As the world's most respected authority on medicine and health, the American Medical Association is committed to helping women live healthy, productive lives. We encourage you to use the information in this book to educate yourself, ask the right questions, work with your doctor, and make informed decisions about your health and health care.

1

Hormones and the Female Reproductive System

To understand menopause and the changes it brings, it is important to have a basic understanding of the body's hormonal, or endocrine, system and the female reproductive system. This information will help you understand more about how your body works, how it changes at menopause, what you can do to minimize the effects, and how various medications work in your body.

WHAT ARE HORMONES?

Hormones are chemical substances produced in the body by organs called endocrine glands. When a hormone is released by an endocrine gland into your bloodstream, it produces an effect in a specific part of the body (sometimes called a "target" organ).

Hormones act as "chemical messengers" that help control and coordinate various body functions, such as metabolism (the way the body turns food into energy), growth and development, sex and reproduction, composition of the blood, reaction to emergencies, and the release of hormones themselves. If the body does not produce the needed amount of each hormone, serious health problems can occur.

The major endocrine glands include the adrenal glands, the pituitary gland, the thyroid gland, the parathyroid glands, and the ovaries.

As the body develops from infancy to adulthood, complex physical changes take place; hormones play a major role in regulating these changes. Puberty, the period of sexual development, begins between ages 10 and 15. At the start of puberty, the hypothalamus (the part of the brain that controls many basic bodily functions, including the endocrine system) secretes more gonadotropin-releasing hormone (GnRH). This hormone stimulates the pituitary gland to secrete follicle-stimulating hormone (FSH) and luteinizing hormone (LH), which are the gonadotropic hormones. These hormones in turn act on the ovaries.

Under the influence of FSH and LH, the ovaries develop and begin to release large amounts of sex hormones into the bloodstream. The female sex hormones are progesterone and estrogen. The adrenal glands also secrete some sex hormones, especially androgens (male sex hormones). The ovaries also secrete some male sex hormones, including testosterone.

The sex hormones control the rapid changes that occur during puberty. For example, they help trigger the increases in height and weight that occur and, at the end of puberty, they help to stop this growth.

ESTROGEN AND PROGESTERONE

The female reproductive system depends primarily on two hormones: estrogen and progesterone. Both are produced in the ovaries. The main role of estrogen and progesterone is to help regulate the menstrual cycle and prepare the uterus for pregnancy. Like all hormones, estrogen and progesterone circulate throughout the body and interact with other hormones and with the body's metabolism. Estrogen affects many tissues throughout the body, including the urethra, bladder, vagina, breasts, bones, skin, liver, arteries, and brain.

When a girl begins puberty, her ovaries start to release increasing amounts of estrogen into her bloodstream. Estrogen stimulates the development of the breasts and causes the genital organs to enlarge and mature. Estrogen also stimulates the endometrium (the lining of the uterus) to thicken.

Estrogen plays an important role in the menstrual cycle and affects almost every part of a woman's body. It influences height and weight, skin tone, muscular strength, digestion, heart rate, and circulation. The ovaries produce varying levels of estrogen throughout a woman's life span. Fat tissues also produce some estrogen.

Estrogen provides several benefits:

- Estrogen helps prevent heart disease by increasing the level of "good" cholesterol in the blood and decreasing the level of "bad" cholesterol, and by keeping coronary arteries open and resistant to plaque (patches of fatty tissue on the inside of arteries) (see Chapter 4).
- Estrogen helps keep breast tissue firm.

- Estrogen helps maintain calcium in the bones, which helps make them dense, strong, and resistant to breaking.
- Estrogen helps keep the vaginal lining moist, keeping it resistant to infection and more comfortable during sexual activity.

Progesterone is produced mainly by the ovaries during a woman's reproductive years and by the placenta during pregnancy. Small amounts are also produced by the adrenal glands.

Progesterone helps prepare the uterus for pregnancy. About midway through a woman's monthly menstrual cycle, one of the two ovaries releases an egg. This process, called ovulation, results in high levels of progesterone being released into the blood for 10 to 12 days. Progesterone stimulates growth of the endometrium (the lining of the uterus) so that the egg, if it has been fertilized, can implant (attach to the uterine wall). If pregnancy does not occur, the ovary stops producing high levels of progesterone. The uterine lining then breaks down and passes out of the body as menstrual fluid.

The increase in progesterone levels after ovulation also causes other cyclic changes. The woman's body temperature increases slightly and her breasts may feel fuller or become sensitive.

MENARCHE

Menarche, or the onset of menstruation, is the result of a series of hormonal changes that take place over the course of several years inside a young girl's body. Before age 8, only small amounts of estrogen are released into the bloodstream. When a girl reaches puberty, her pituitary gland begins to produce the hormones that are vital to sexual development. One of them is FSH (follicle-stimulating hormone), which will play an important part in the reproductive cycle. Another hormone, growth hormone, accelerates body growth, causing the typical "growth spurt" of the teenage years.

As puberty continues, the pituitary gland produces more FSH, causing the ovaries to produce estrogen. The higher level of estrogen in the bloodstream causes the development of female sex characteristics in classic sequence: first, the breasts develop and pubic hair begins to grow; then, underarm hair appears and menstruation begins; and finally, the hips begin to broaden, producing the characteristic female shape.

Estrogen also produces other changes in the body. By closing the ends of the bones, it stops skeletal growth. Generally, girls stop growing in height one or two years after menstruation begins. Estrogen also causes fat to be deposited in the labia, making them thicker. Pubic hair becomes denser and coarser in texture. The clitoris enlarges and becomes more sensitive. The vagina increases in length, and growth occurs in the uterus, fallopian tubes, and ovaries. Finally, as the body, brain, and endocrine glands mature, menstruation begins.

The first menstrual period usually occurs between ages 11 to 14, but this varies widely. It may be influenced by diet, exercise, genetics, and other factors. Ovulation is rare during the first year of menstrual cycles, which are often irregular, and sometimes heavy.

MENSTRUATION

The female reproductive system (see illustration) consists of the ovaries, fallopian tubes, uterus, and vagina. At birth, a female infant has about 2 million eggs (or ova) in her ovaries. By puberty, the ovaries contain just 300,000 eggs, each surrounded by a casing of cells called a follicle.

During a woman's reproductive years, about 450 eggs reach maturity and travel through the fallopian tubes, where they can be fertilized by sperm. The rest of the eggs slowly disintegrate, and by menopause, only about 3,000 remain.

As mentioned above, menstrual cycles (see illustration) depend on the interrelationships and functioning of the various endocrine glands. Menstruation is initially triggered by hormones released from the hypothalamus. At puberty, the hypothalamus begins to release GnRH (gonadotropin-releasing hormone), which signals to the pituitary gland to secrete FSH (follicle-stimulating hormone) and LH (luteinizing hormone). These two hormones act on the ovaries and help coordinate the menstrual cycle.

In the first phase of the menstrual cycle, called the proliferative phase, the pituitary gland releases more FSH than LH. When FSH reaches the ovaries, it causes one of the follicles to grow and secrete estrogen. When the amount of estrogen in the bloodstream reaches a certain level, it stimulates the pituitary gland to secrete more LH. Then the egg is mature and ready to leave the follicle. The follicle ruptures and the egg is released from the ovary. This is known as ovulation, and it occurs 14 days before the next menstruation, regardless of the length of the cycle, or at the halfway point of a 28-day menstrual cycle. The egg passes into the fallopian tube, where it can be fertilized if sperm are present.

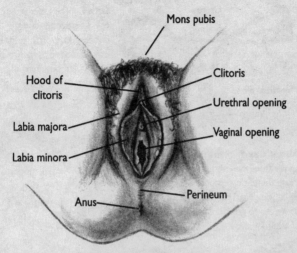

External female genitalia

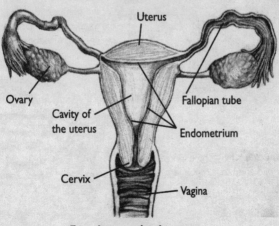

Female reproductive organs

The menstrual cycle

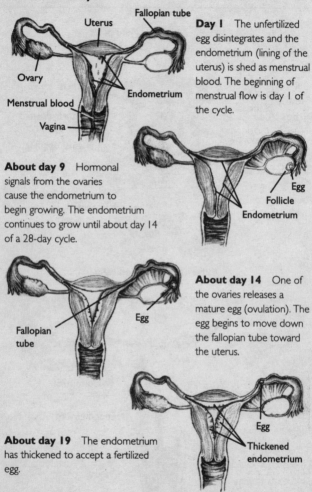

Day 1 The unfertilized egg disintegrates and the endometrium (lining of the uterus) is shed as menstrual blood. The beginning of menstrual flow is day 1 of the cycle.

Uterus
Fallopian tube
Ovary
Endometrium
Menstrual blood
Vagina

About day 9 Hormonal signals from the ovaries cause the endometrium to begin growing. The endometrium continues to grow until about day 14 of a 28-day cycle.

Egg
Follicle
Endometrium

About day 14 One of the ovaries releases a mature egg (ovulation). The egg begins to move down the fallopian tube toward the uterus.

Fallopian tube
Egg

About day 19 The endometrium has thickened to accept a fertilized egg.

Egg
Thickened endometrium

In the second, or luteal, phase of the menstrual cycle, the cells that lined the follicle from which the egg was released are transformed into the corpus luteum. Beginning just hours after ovulation, the corpus luteum secretes small amounts of estrogen and large amounts of progesterone to help thicken the endometrium (lining of the uterus). The corpus luteum also produces inhibin, a hormone that, along with estrogen and progesterone, signals the pituitary to stop secreting FSH and LH. As a result, the amount of both FSH and LH in the blood falls to low levels.

If the egg is fertilized by a sperm, it implants in the uterus and secretes a hormone called human chorionic gonadotropin (HCG). This hormone stimulates the continued secretion of estrogen and progesterone so that the developing embryo will be nourished.

If the egg is not fertilized, the corpus luteum disintegrates and estrogen and progesterone secretion decreases. The sudden drop in blood levels of these two hormones, in turn, causes the endometrium to break down. A day or two later, the uterine lining is shed and menstruation begins. Periods, on average, last from 3 to 7 days.

During menstruation, the pituitary gland starts secreting FSH and LH again, stimulating the development of another follicle and beginning the menstrual cycle over again. In general, the entire cycle takes about 28 days, but no woman is always regular; cycles as short as 21 days or as long as 35 days are not uncommon—even in the same woman.

During the days before a menstrual cycle begins, some women have emotional or physical symptoms that may include mood swings, anxiety, fatigue, irritability, headache, swelling, and/or breast tenderness. This condition is often referred to as premenstrual syndrome (PMS). According to research, PMS seems to result from hormone fluctuations. One treatment for PMS is the birth control pill, because it provides a steady, daily dose of hormones that does not fluctuate.

In addition to PMS, some women have discomfort or cramps as the uterus contracts during menstruation. This discomfort or pain, called dysmenorrhea, varies from woman to woman and from month to month. The discomfort and pain of PMS can be treated with nonsteroidal anti-inflammatory drugs (NSAIDs), such as ibuprofen. Talk to your doctor if you have symptoms of PMS or discomfort or cramps during menstruation.

By the time a woman reaches her mid- to late thirties, the number of follicles in her ovaries has gradually declined. At about the same time, the remaining follicles become less responsive to FSH and LH. As a result, the ovaries produce less and less estrogen and progesterone. In response, the pituitary gland secretes higher levels of FSH and LH to stimulate the ovaries.

Initially, a woman may not notice any difference in her menstrual cycles. But between 2 and 8 years before menopause, her menstrual flow will change. It may become heavier one month, lighter the next, and she may even miss periods altogether. This transition period is commonly referred to as perimenopause. As the levels of estrogen and progesterone produced by the ovaries drop, menstruation stops completely. This is known as menopause and occurs at an average age of 51.

2

The Arrival of Menopause

Most women go through menopause with few problems. Some even look forward to menopause because they will no longer need to worry about getting pregnant or having monthly periods.

PERIMENOPAUSE (PREMENOPAUSE)

Women in their late thirties to midforties may begin to notice changes in their menstrual cycles; some may begin to have hot flashes. Many of these women may think that they have reached menopause. It is important to note, however, that these symptoms are more likely perimenopause, the months or years that make up the transition period that leads up to menopause.

Symptoms of perimenopause usually begin in a woman's forties. For most women, perimenopause begins 2 or 3 years before their final menstrual period, which for the average American woman occurs around age 51. Menopause occurs when the ovaries no longer produce enough estrogen to sustain full menstrual cycles.

As with the menstrual cycle and menopause in general, the effects of menopause vary from woman to woman and from month to month. An irregular menstrual cycle is usually the first sign of perimenopause. This irregularity may take the form of missed periods, longer intervals between periods, irregular bleeding, varying lengths of periods, or a decrease or increase in menstrual flow. These changes may be different from month to month. Symptoms related to perimenopause include hot flashes, night sweats, insomnia, mood swings, and vaginal dryness. Most of these physical and emotional symptoms are directly caused by lowered levels of estrogen. Other factors, such as lifestyle, stress, and major life changes, can play an important role.

It is important to note that perimenopause occurs at a time in life when pelvic disorders are common. This means that irregular bleeding is not always related to menopause. It could be a symptom of another medical problem. Heavy bleeding, for example, may indicate the presence of fibroids (noncancerous tumors) in the uterus, endometrial polyps, precancerous conditions, or cancer. For this reason, it is important to report any menstrual irregularities to your doctor. Similarly, if you stop menstruating (a condition known as amenorrhea), it does not always mean that you have reached menopause. You could be pregnant or have thyroid or adrenal gland problems. Again, report any significant changes in your menstrual cycle to your doctor.

Women who have ovaries typically begin perimenopause gradually. Perimenopause typically lasts about 4 to 6 years. But some women may skip perimenopause altogether.

Some women get relief from the symptoms of perimenopause by taking low-dose oral contraceptives (birth control pills), as prescribed by their doctors. These pills provide a woman with a daily dose of estrogen and progesterone. This prevents hormone levels from fluctuating, and a woman continues to get her monthly menstrual period. For information on how to deal with the specific symptoms of perimenopause and menopause, read Chapter 3.

MENOPAUSE

Menopause is the stage of life when a woman stops menstruating. It marks the natural end of a woman's reproductive years. And while perimenopause can last for months or years, menopause usually occurs quickly, with the last menstrual period. Menopause often follows hereditary patterns; a woman is likely to go through menopause at the same age as her mother.

Attitudes toward menopause vary from one culture to another. In western culture, because there is strong emphasis on female youth and beauty, menopause is often viewed as a time of decline and loss of status for women. Therefore, it is not surprising that many American women have a negative view of menopause. Other societies view menopause in a more positive light, giving older women increased status in the family and greater freedom in society.

OTHER REASONS FOR MENOPAUSE

Menopause does not always happen naturally, and sometimes women reach menopause at a time that differs greatly from that of the "average" woman.

Premature Menopause

Premature menopause, stopping menstruation before age 40, is uncommon. It occurs when the ovaries stop functioning at an early age. When menopause does occur early, there is often a family history of premature menopause or health problems that can cause early menopause. (Women who smoke tend to reach menopause 1 or 2 years earlier than women who do not smoke, but rarely before age 40.)

If a woman under age 40 stops having menstrual periods, there are many possible causes. Pregnancy, stress, and illness are common causes. Another possible cause is anorexia nervosa, a life-threatening eating disorder. Weight loss and prolonged strenuous exercise can also play a role. Stopping oral contraceptives may cause periods to stop temporarily for several months. Occasionally, an excess of prolactin, the milk-promoting hormone of the pituitary gland, or a pituitary tumor interrupts menstrual periods. Also, some drugs prescribed to treat severe depression may cause a woman's periods to stop.

Each of these possibilities needs to be considered when a woman's periods prematurely stop. The follicle-stimulating hormone (FSH) blood test used to determine menopause can also be used to diagnose premature menopause. Once the cause of the amenorrhea is determined, the underlying problem can be treated. Then, when the woman's general health, emotional well-being, or hormone balance improves, the pituitary gland will usually secrete FSH and luteinizing hormone (LH) again, stimulating the ovaries to produce estrogen and allowing menstrual periods to resume.

If you think you may have premature menopause, early diagnosis is important so that you can begin hormone replacement therapy (HRT). Women who have early menopause may live for many years without estrogen's positive effects on their bones and cardiovascular system (the heart and blood vessels). Therefore, these women have an increased risk for both heart disease and the debilitating bone disease known as osteoporosis. If you are in your twenties or thirties and have stopped menstruating, see your doctor as soon as possible.

Premature menopause can be especially difficult for women who want to have children. However, with advances in reproductive technology, it is now possible for these women to try to become pregnant. By using hormone treatment and eggs from a donor, postmenopausal women, particularly those under age 45, may still be able to become pregnant.

Late Menopause

Late menopause (when menstruation continues past age 54) also tends to be hereditary. In addition, women with diabetes often have late menopause. Although it is not uncommon to have regular periods up to age 53, very few women continue to menstruate after this age. Some doctors believe that women who have late menopause are at greater risk for cancer of the uterus or breast cancer.

If you are in your midfifties and still have vaginal bleeding, do not automatically assume that you are still having "normal" menstruation. Vaginal bleeding at this age can be a symptom of a serious health problem. If you continue to have any vaginal bleeding after your 53rd birthday, see your doctor without delay. For more information about abnormal vaginal bleeding, read Chapter 9.

Surgical Menopause

Surgical menopause occurs when a woman has a hysterectomy in which her ovaries are removed along with her uterus. Removal of the ovaries results in the sudden loss of estrogen and usually causes immediate menopausal symptoms.

If the ovaries are not removed during a hysterectomy, they continue to function until a woman's natural age of menopause. Surgical removal of one ovary does not affect the body's estrogen levels, since the remaining ovary supplies enough estrogen to suppress menopausal symptoms.

For some women, surgical menopause may be more difficult than natural menopause, because symptoms such as hot flashes and vaginal dryness appear suddenly and may be frequent and severe. However, these symptoms can be effectively treated with hormone replacement.

Estrogen also has a positive effect on cholesterol levels; it increases the level of high density lipoprotein (HDL, or "good") cholesterol in the bloodstream and decreases the level of low density lipoprotein (LDL, or "bad") cholesterol. When the ovaries are removed and natural estrogen levels drop, this benefit is lost. Therefore, a woman whose ovaries are removed before natural menopause occurs has a higher risk of developing heart disease later on in life. However, replacing the estrogen that the woman's body is no longer producing maintains her protection against heart disease.

Temporary Menopause

When women in their reproductive years take chemotherapy for cancer, they may begin to miss menstrual periods and develop menopausal symptoms.

Certain types of chemotherapy produce temporary menopause because the drugs used affect the ripening eggs inside the ovaries. The effect of chemotherapy varies with age and with the dose and type of treatment given. Women under 35 may regain their periods and fertility when the chemotherapy treatments are stopped, but women over 35 to 40 often remain menopausal. Radiation to the ovaries can affect their function, resulting in premature ovarian failure and menopause.

If a woman's cancer is not estrogen related, she is usually given hormone therapy, including estrogen, for the symptoms of early menopause. Estrogen-related cancers include breast cancer and endometrial cancer. Women with breast cancer are usually advised not to use estrogen. Women with endometrial cancer, however, are sometimes offered HRT if their cancer has been diagnosed and treated at an early stage and shows no sign of recurrence.

IDENTIFYING MENOPAUSE

It is difficult to predict when a woman will reach menopause. Both physical characteristics and heredity play a role. For example, obese women tend to reach menopause later in life than thin women. As we have noted, there also is a tendency for daughters to follow the menstrual pattern of their mothers. There is no relationship, however, between the age of menarche (the onset of menstruation) and that of menopause. Nor does the number of children a woman has or the age at which she first engages in sexual activity affect when she reaches menopause.

If you are having irregular menstrual periods, a blood test to measure FSH (follicle-stimulating hormone) is the best indicator of menopause. As your estrogen level drops, the pituitary gland secretes more FSH in an effort to stimulate the ovaries to produce more estrogen. Your level of FSH will help your doctor determine whether you are at or approaching menopause.

For many women, the symptoms of menopause are obvious and an FSH test is completely unnecessary. However, the test can be useful if the cause of missed periods is in question, especially in a younger woman. It is also helpful in women who have had a hysterectomy and are unable to rely on menstrual periods as an indicator of menopause. Also, FSH testing is the only way for women who take oral contraceptives to know whether they have reached menopause.

Along with the results of the FSH blood test, the following are signs that can help you determine if you are approaching menopause:

- Your menstrual cycles are irregular and have been for several months, or you have missed some periods.

- You have awakened at night drenched in sweat. (This sensation is known as a night sweat.)
- You are having hot flashes—brief episodes of intense heat and flushing felt especially on the head, neck, and upper chest.

3

Symptoms of Menopause

While many women may believe that menopause causes a specific group of symptoms that all women will experience, this is not true. Each woman's experience with menopause is unique. In fact, the only symptom that all women going through menopause share is the end of menstrual periods. But how and when they end varies.

Identifying the possible symptoms of menopause is complicated by the fact that menopause usually occurs when the body is undergoing changes related to normal aging, such as wrinkles, stiff joints, and brittle bones. Because menopause and age-related changes occur around the same time, some women may think that menopause causes these changes. Aging is influenced by a number of factors, including genetics, diet, hormones, physical activity, stress, history of injury and disease, and medications. But by taking good care of yourself, particularly in your middle years, you can slow many of the changes that occur as you grow older.

Research has shown that estrogen has a strong influence on blood-cholesterol levels and bone mass. Lower estrogen levels after menopause often raise low density lipoprotein (LDL)-cholesterol (the "bad" cholesterol) levels, which is one reason women have an increased risk of developing heart disease in their later years. Estrogen also protects a woman's bone mass. The drop in estrogen levels after menopause speeds bone loss, which increases a woman's risk of developing osteoporosis and the debilitating bone fractures that come with it. However, you can reduce the risks of these menopause-related changes by living a healthy lifestyle and by taking hormone replacement therapy (HRT), which can slow the effects of aging on your heart, bones, brain, vagina, and breasts. For more information about HRT, read Chapter 5. For more information on a healthy lifestyle, read Chapter 7.

The following section describes the most common symptoms of perimenopause and menopause, their causes, and steps you can take to prevent or relieve these symptoms.

IRREGULAR MENSTRUAL CYCLES

The most common symptom of perimenopause is irregular menstrual cycles. Shorter or longer periods, heavier or lighter menstrual flow, and varying lengths of time between periods indicate that perimenopause has begun and menopause is approaching. Unpredictability is usually the main inconvenience of irregular cycles.

Causes

As menopause nears, many women experience changes in their menstrual cycle. Periods usually become farther apart and menstrual flow becomes lighter. If menstruation does not occur for 12 months, menopause probably has occurred. If you have vaginal bleeding after 1 year without a menstrual period, see your doctor as soon as possible; bleeding after menopause may be a symptom of abnormal tissue inside the uterus.

For other women, irregular periods are accompanied by heavy bleeding. If ovulation does not occur on a regular basis, not enough progesterone is produced to balance the effect of estrogen on the uterine lining. The excess estrogen causes the endometrium to build up, eventually resulting in a heavy flow, sometimes with clots. Heavy periods such as these can be painful.

What to Do

Once medical problems such as abnormal tissue inside the uterus or fibroids are ruled out, there are a number of useful options for dealing with the inconvenience of irregular menstrual cycles.

One method is to keep track of your cycles with a diary. This helps you to recognize overall patterns in your cycles, so you can know better what to expect. It also provides you with valuable information your doctor can use to help determine treatment. In your diary, note the beginning and end of your cycle, the type of flow, and any symptoms—such as cramps—that occur. Also note bleeding that occurs at any time other than at the end of your monthly cycle.

Some women get relief from irregular menstrual bleeding by taking oral contraceptives, which help to regulate the menstrual cycle until menopause arrives. Other benefits of oral contraceptives are particularly important for perimenopausal women, such as protection against endometrial cancer and breast cancer.

It is especially important for a woman to maintain a healthy diet (see page 132) during this stage of her life. For many women with heavy or frequent menstrual periods, iron deficiency anemia results from the increased blood loss. Getting plenty of iron in your diet can help offset this loss. Good sources of iron include beef, poultry, prunes, raisins, and spinach. Some women may need to take an iron supplement. Also, extra vitamin C may be useful, because it helps your body absorb iron. Good sources of vitamin C include citrus fruits, blueberries, grapes, and cherries.

For many women in their forties and fifties, irregular bleeding is not always a symptom of perimenopause. Instead, it may be a symptom of a gynecologic or other health disorder. Many health problems can cause irregular menstrual flow, including thyroid disorders and uterine conditions, such as fibroids, polyps, and precancerous or cancerous growths, and hormonal abnormalities, such as failure to ovulate. If you experience irregular bleeding, especially if it is accompanied by pain and discomfort, urinary or bowel changes, fatigue, or other unusual symptoms, consult your doctor without delay.

HOT FLASHES

Hot flashes are a common symptom of perimenopause and menopause. They are often one of the earliest indicators of approaching menopause, sometimes beginning several years ahead of other symptoms.

More than 50 percent of women get hot flashes or other symptoms such as dizziness and heart palpitations. The sensation produced by hot flashes varies from woman to woman and from one episode to another. In general, hot flashes cause a sudden feeling of warmth throughout the upper body or over the entire body. This sudden wave of heat typically starts in the upper chest and neck and spreads upward to the face and down the shoulders. It is often followed by flushing, perspiration, and a cold, clammy sensation as the body temperature readjusts. A hot flash may last anywhere from a few seconds to a few minutes.

For some women, hot flashes are little more than a slightly noticeable sensation of warmth. Others may experience waves of heat, drenching sweats, and a rapid heartbeat. Hot flashes may occur several times a day, once a week, or only occasionally. Initially, they are common at night or at times of stress. Poor sleeping patterns can lead to fatigue, irritability, poor concentration, and forgetfulness.

Women who have their ovaries removed as part of a hysterectomy and do not take HRT tend to have more severe hot flashes than women who go through natural menopause, at least for the first year after the surgery. This is because the drop in estrogen levels among these women is so abrupt.

Causes

Hot flashes are caused by the pituitary gland's response to declining estrogen levels. The pituitary responds by increasing its secretion of luteinizing hormone (LH) in sudden bursts. These LH surges cause the sudden temperature rises, or "flashes."

No two women experience hot flashes in exactly the same

way. Some women never experience them at all, while others have them only occasionally. Obese women are less troubled by hot flashes. This is probably because their own natural androgens are converted into estrogens by enzymes in their body fat.

Treatment

Here are a number of self-help measures you can use to deal with hot flashes:

• **Keep a diary of your hot flashes.** Hot flashes do not always take you by surprise. There are certain things that can trigger them, including hot weather, caffeine, or stress. When you keep track of your hot flashes for a week or two, you may discover those things that trigger them. This information will help you to manage your hot flashes.

• **Dress in layers.** Wear layers of clothing that can be easily removed during a hot flash. Clothes made of natural fibers are best because they absorb moisture, dry quickly, and allow heat to escape.

• **Keep cool.** Wherever you spend a lot of time—at home or at your office—do what you can to keep cool. Set your thermostat to a comfortable temperature. Keep an electric or hand-held fan close by. Sit next to the air conditioner or away from heat ducts at meetings or social gatherings. To reduce night sweats, keep your bedroom cool, open windows, and use an air conditioner in the summer.

• **Avoid stressful situations.** Stress can trigger hot flashes. For help in avoiding or handling stress, see Chapter 7.

• **Cool off with water.** Run cold water over your wrists or splash water on your face to cool off. If possible, take a cool shower.

• **Perform deep-breathing exercises.** If stress triggers hot flashes for you, deep-breathing exercises (see page 177) may help alleviate them.

• **Watch your diet.** Reduce the number of empty calories you consume each day. Fatty foods and alcohol are common sources of such calories. These and other foods may trigger hot flashes. While keeping your hot flash diary, be sure to note all the foods you eat each day and watch for those that seem to trigger hot flashes.

• **Try a vitamin E supplement, if your doctor approves.** Many women find relief from hot flashes with vitamin E. Good sources of vitamin E include vegetable oils, nuts, whole grains, and wheat germ. Alternative practitioners think that large doses of vitamin E (from 800 to 1,600 international units a day) help relieve hot flashes and other symptoms of menopause. However, mainstream medicine does not endorse this, and there is no research verifying that it is safe to take such large doses. Ask your doctor how much of the vitamin you need to take each day.

• **Consider hormone replacement therapy.** Even if your hot flashes are not severe, ask your doctor about HRT. Estrogen replacement is the most effective method for controlling hot flashes. Read Chapter 5 for more information about HRT and whether you should take it.

• **Ask your doctor about other prescription medications.** There are nonhormonal prescription medications available if you cannot take HRT. These drugs, such as clonidine, are often effective in reducing hot flashes. For more information about drugs used for the symptoms of menopause, read Chapter 6.

VAGINAL DRYNESS

Because estrogen plays such an important role in a woman's reproductive system, the decline in estrogen at menopause brings significant changes in all the reproductive organs. Some women begin to experience vaginal problems during perimenopause, but for most, these problems do not occur until one or more years after menopause. At that time, the lining of the vagina usually becomes thinner, less elastic, and drier, and over time, the vagina shrinks. Burning and itching sensations may accompany the vaginal dryness, which can be aggravated by reduced secretion of cervical mucus. All of these factors can cause pain or bleeding during intercourse. Do not hesitate to talk to your doctor about any vaginal irritation or painful intercourse.

Here are some methods of dealing with vaginal dryness:

• **Stay sexually active.** As with any other muscle in your body, lack of use of the vaginal muscle results in diminished tone and decreased flexibility. Without use, eventually the vaginal muscle will shrink. If you have a regular sex partner, your doctor will probably recommend regular intercourse to aid in continuing lubrication, muscle tone, and sexual health. Women who engage in sexual activity at least once a week maintain better vaginal health than those who do not.

Sexual arousal produces some natural lubrication by increasing blood flow to the vagina. This helps in the secretion of lubricating fluid through the vaginal lining. Any sexual activity—including masturbation—helps improve blood flow to the vagina and keeps tissues supple.

• **Perform Kegel exercises.** Kegel exercises strengthen the muscles of the pelvic floor. They are the most popular exercises for this purpose. As with all exercises, the more diligently you perform them, the greater the benefit.

To practice doing Kegel exercises, try to stop the flow of your urine the next time you go to the bathroom. Stopping the flow of urine indicates to you exactly where these muscles are. Then you can practice this exercise for multiple repetitions. The best part about working these muscles is that you do not have to strain to benefit and you can do the exercises anytime, anywhere. Breathe naturally as you do these exercises.

Begin exercising your pelvic floor muscles by contracting (tightening) hard for a second and then releasing completely. Repeat this ten times to make up one set of exercises. In a month's time, try to work up to 20 sets during one day. You can do this at any time—while sitting in a car or bus, while waiting in line at the grocery store, while talking on the telephone, or while taking a shower.

Ideally, you should have begun performing Kegel exercises while in your teens. And if you have been diligent, you have been doing them ever since. If you have ever been pregnant, chances are your doctor encouraged you to do these exercises to help prepare the muscles for childbirth and to help them recover from a vaginal birth. Kegel exercises can improve sexual satisfaction and are useful for women of any age who have urinary incontinence.

• **Use a lubricant.** Some women find that using a water-based lubricant during intercourse helps to alleviate the problems associated with vaginal dryness. Oil-based products, such as petroleum jelly and baby oil, should not be used, because they tend to coat the vaginal lining and inhibit your own natural secretions.

INSOMNIA

A major problem for women with hot flashes is that their sleep can be disrupted. Many, but not all, of these sleep problems are the result of hot flashes. Stress, diet, and medications can all disrupt sleep.

Here are some steps you can take to ensure a better night's sleep:

- **Avoid sleep medications.** Some doctors may recommend occasional use of sleeping medications for symptom relief. However, over-the-counter or prescription sleep medications do nothing to treat the underlying problem of menopause-related insomnia. Health experts generally recommend that you try to avoid these sleep aids. For occasional insomnia, first try to improve your sleep habits. A few suggestions follow.
- **Keep to a sleep schedule.** Go to bed and wake up at the same times each day.
- **Control your sleep environment.** Sleep in a dark room or use an eye covering. Block out noise as best you can. Keep your bedroom cool and comfortable.
- **Exercise regularly.** Daily workouts tire out the body and prepare it for a good night's sleep. Do not exercise too close to bedtime, however. Late-night workouts can overstimulate your body, contributing to insomnia.
- **Avoid caffeinated drinks and foods late in the day.** If you are having trouble sleeping, avoid coffee, tea, caffeinated soft drinks, chocolate, and other caffeinated foods in the late afternoon or evening. If you are having problems with frequent urination at night, decrease the amount of fluids you drink in the evening.

• **Watch your diet.** The types, amounts, and timing of foods and drinks may prevent you from falling asleep or may awaken you during the night. A diet high in fat, caffeine, and alcohol can alter sleep patterns. For example, eating a large, heavy, fatty meal too close to bedtime can keep you awake for hours. The caffeine in coffee, chocolate, soda, and tea can also interfere with a good night's sleep. You should also avoid drinking too much alcohol. While you may fall asleep quickly after consuming alcohol, it can cause you to awaken several times during the night.

And finally, as you age, you become more susceptible to the effects of heartburn. An unsettled stomach can awaken you and make it difficult to fall back to sleep. Keep track of the foods that seem to give you heartburn and avoid them, especially close to bedtime. Take an antacid tablet or acid blocker before bedtime to help prevent the problem. Some antacids have the added benefit of calcium, a mineral that all women need.

• **Relax before bedtime.** A hot bath or relaxation exercises may bring about better sleep. Allow some time to read, watch television, or write before heading to bed. If you find you cannot sleep once you are in bed, do not try too hard to fall asleep. Instead, get up and try some more relaxing activities, such as light reading or simple chores.

• **Ask about hormone replacement therapy.** Even if your insomnia is not so severe that it interferes with your daily living, ask your doctor about the effects of HRT on sleeplessness. HRT can be very effective in combating insomnia. Women who take estrogen generally fall asleep faster, sleep longer, have fewer episodes of wakefulness, and have more periods of beneficial REM (rapid eye movement, or dream) sleep than women who do not take estrogen.

As with many symptoms of menopause, there are other causes of insomnia. If you have frequent problems with sleep, talk to your doctor.

EMOTIONAL SYMPTOMS

Forgetfulness, lack of concentration, anxiety, irritability, and depressed mood are all common emotional symptoms of women who are going through or have reached menopause. In most instances, these symptoms are related to estrogen deficiency.

There is no overall increased incidence of depression among postmenopausal women. And while some women may be depressed or have regrets about losing their ability to bear children, this is often balanced by feelings of relief that they do not have to worry about contraception or menstrual periods. However, many women will experience emotional ups and downs related to the hormonal changes of menopause. It is important to point out, however, that irritability, impaired memory, and anxiety are classic symptoms of chronic sleep disturbances. As we have mentioned, hot flashes and night sweats, which are caused by hormones, often disrupt sleep. Therefore, if you have insomnia or other sleep disturbances, your emotional symptoms may be relieved as soon as you can resolve your sleep problems.

How do hormones influence your mood? Estrogen affects the brain and central nervous system. As estrogen decreases, levels of endorphins (chemicals in the brain that make you feel good) also fall. When the drop is sudden, as following a hysterectomy, chances of extreme mood disturbances increase. Immediate HRT is highly successful in these women.

Of course, hormones will not completely help women who have clinical depression or other serious psychological problems. Also, stress or problems with everyday life at this stage of life could trigger bouts of insomnia, irritability, depression, and mood swings, which cannot be fully helped with hormones. Stress may also result in episodes of anxiety or even "panic attacks."

Menopause is also a reminder that you are aging. Your attitude toward aging may influence the way you feel and may increase your anxiety. Your partner's feelings about your menopause can also influence how you feel.

A key to relieving your anxiety is to gain an understanding of the physical changes you are going through. Learn as much as you can about menopause, aging, osteoporosis, and other related topics of interest to you. Keep the lines of communication open with those people who mean the most to you, including your partner and children, if any. Individual or group counseling may also be beneficial.

CHANGES IN LIBIDO

Menopause does not mean the end of sex. In fact, for many women, menopause is the time when they are most sexually satisfied and creative. This may be due in part to the fact that there is no longer the fear of an unintended pregnancy and the need for birth control devices. In addition, some of the hormonal changes women experience at menopause actually heighten sexual response.

A woman's libido seems to depend on a number of factors,

such as genetics, upbringing, and life experiences. Sex drive is predominantly psychological, but there are some physical changes that may alter it.

The changes that take place in the vagina and in hormonal secretions at menopause may cause a temporary decline in a woman's sexual responsiveness. The stopping of menstrual periods and declining levels of female hormones, however, do not directly affect sexual desire. In fact, a woman's sexual interest and enjoyment do not necessarily decrease at midlife, but may actually increase. This is because of the change in the ratio of male to female hormones.

The hormone most responsible for sexual arousal is the male hormone testosterone. While testosterone is present in a woman's bloodstream prior to menopause, its effect is tempered by the larger proportions of estrogen and progesterone. As the levels of these female hormones fall at menopause, the proportion of testosterone rises, thereby increasing a woman's sexual interest and enjoyment. Decreased libido may be more common in surgical menopause because removal of the ovaries also decreases testosterone levels.

OTHER BODY CHANGES

Estrogen has a number of significant effects on a woman's physical health and emotional well-being. Estrogen acts directly on the uterus and affects other organs and tissues such as the vulva, vagina, breasts, bones, heart, central nervous system, hair, and skin. As the level of estrogen decreases, major changes occur in the appearance and function of all of these organs. But not every menopausal symptom is caused by declining hormones. Some of these changes are the natural results of aging.

Postmenopausal women who do not take HRT will experience varying degrees of changes in the vagina, cervix, uterus, and ovaries. Along with detecting a decrease in the size of the cervix and uterus, many women notice a reduction in cervical mucus and vaginal lubrication. Without estrogen, the acid-base balance of the vagina changes, and women become more prone to bacterial infections. The labia majora, the larger outer skin folds of the vagina, become thinner, flatter, paler, and less elastic. The vaginal walls thin, and the vagina shortens and loses its elasticity and muscle tone, as well as some of its normal secretions, sometimes making intercourse uncomfortable or painful.

The pelvic-floor muscles, which support the pelvic organs, including the bladder and urethra, can lose muscle tone as a result of low levels of estrogen after menopause. Lack of muscle tone may cause the urethra to sag, so that a small amount of urine escapes when pressure inside the abdomen increases and other organs press on the bladder. This involuntary leaking of urine, called stress incontinence, can occur when you sneeze, cough, or perform such high-impact exercises as jogging.

Urge incontinence is the involuntary leaking of urine after a sudden, overwhelming urge to urinate, even though the bladder may contain very little urine. It is caused by involuntary contraction of the bladder muscle. The cause of these contractions is usually unknown, but they are more common after menopause.

Urinary incontinence can be greatly alleviated by HRT. Kegel exercises (see page 29) may also strengthen the pelvic-floor muscles. Because these muscles support the vaginal tissues and blad-

PHYSICAL CHANGES AT MENOPAUSE

- Some shrinking of the vagina, cervix, uterus, and ovaries
- Shortening of the vagina, with loss of muscle tone and thinning of the lining
- Changes in labia majora including possible thinning, paleness, and loss of elasticity
- Loss of muscle tone of supporting ligaments
- Reduction in vaginal and cervical secretions
- Changes in breast size, firmness, and shape
- Thinning of body hair in most women; possible increase of facial hair
- Wrinkling and loss of skin tone
- Loss of bone mass
- Slowing of metabolic rate

der as well as the internal pelvic organs, all benefit from strengthening. Urge incontinence may be helped by bladder training (see page 209). Talk to your doctor about your treatment options.

The breasts also change around menopause. The amount of fat within the breasts increases, altering their size, shape, and firmness. Nipples tend to become smaller and less erect. Estrogen therapy usually replaces most of the fullness in the breast tissue.

Aging also creates changes in the hair and skin. Body hair may thin in some women and increase in others. New growth on the upper lip and chin is due to the reversed ratio of estrogen to androgens (male sex hormones). Wrinkling and loss of skin tone occur most frequently around the face, neck, and hands. Wrinkles may form around the mouth and at the corners of the eyes. Preventive measures, such as wearing sunglasses or a hat with a brim and using sunblock, can minimize some fine aging lines.

If they are not taking HRT, some women are prone to urinary

tract infections around the time of menopause. This is because of the thinning of the tissues in and around the vagina, which are more susceptible to trauma and bacteria. These bladder infections tend to recur but are usually easily treated with antibiotics. Preventive techniques include estrogen vaginal cream to nourish the tissues, urinating after intercourse to rinse bacteria out of the urethra, drinking adequate amounts of fluids, and keeping the genital area very clean. Symptoms include painful or frequent urination.

4

Health Risks of Menopause

Because estrogen plays such an important role, affecting not just a woman's reproductive cycle but her entire body, the declining levels of this hormone around the time of menopause have some dramatic effects on her health. A woman is at higher risk for heart disease, osteoporosis, and other life-threatening diseases after she reaches menopause. This chapter takes a closer look at the health risks that accompany menopause.

HEART DISEASE AND MENOPAUSE

Estrogen protects women against heart disease during the pre-menopausal years. The loss of this hormone at menopause significantly increases a woman's risk of heart disease.

While often thought of as a disease that affects mostly men, heart disease is also a serious problem for women. One in nine women between ages 45 and 64 has some form of cardiovascular disease. Half of all women will eventually die of heart disease.

Heart disease is the leading cause of death for American women. Women tend to develop heart disease about 10 years later than men because estrogen protects women earlier in life. Since many people assume women are less likely to have a heart attack, chest pain and other symptoms of heart disease are often misinterpreted. When heart disease is correctly diagnosed in women, it is often treated less aggressively than it is in men.

Your risk of developing heart disease depends on several factors. But by making certain lifestyle changes now, you may be able to avoid this life-threatening disease in the future.

Types of Heart Disease

The most common and dangerous form of heart disease is ischemic heart disease, which results from injury to the blood vessels that supply the heart muscle, thus obstructing the flow of blood, oxygen, and nutrients. As people age, the diameter of the coronary arteries narrows because of the buildup of artery-clogging plaque (patches of fatty tissue on the inside lining of arteries). This plaque penetrates into the layers of the arterial wall and hardens there, blocking the flow of blood through the vessel. This obstruction is known as atherosclerosis.

Because blood is forced through an increasingly narrow channel, blood flow to the heart declines, leaving the heart starved for oxygen and causing a type of pain called angina. If a blood clot that has formed in a larger blood vessel in another part of the body floats through the coronary artery system, it may become lodged in the smaller coronary artery and block it. As a result of this blocked circulation, a part of the heart muscle will die. This is called myocardial infarction (MI), or heart attack. A blockage is not the only cause of a heart attack, however. Sometimes the wall of the artery contracts, causing the artery to go into spasm. A sudden, prolonged spasm can lead to a heart attack. This explains why young women who do not have significant atherosclerosis can still have heart attacks, although they are uncommon in women under age 50.

Angina is chest pain that occurs when the heart receives an inadequate blood supply during periods of increased demand, such as strenuous exercise or emotional excitement. During such periods, the coronary arteries ordinarily dilate (widen) to deliver more blood and oxygen to the heart muscle. Arteries clogged with plaque, however, gradually become rigid, fail to dilate, and cannot meet the heart's demand for more blood.

In the past, angina in women was often dismissed as something benign, perhaps related to anxiety, and not requiring further follow-up by doctors. Today, both women and their doctors know that chest pain can be a symptom of heart disease and that it should never be ignored.

Silent or unrecognized MI (a heart attack without symptoms) has been found to be more common in women than in men. Studies have also shown that in contrast to a man's first heart attack, a woman's first heart attack is more likely to be fatal; a woman will require longer hospitalization afterward, and she is more likely to die in the first year following the heart attack.

Atherosclerosis is a progressive problem that can begin early

---

WARNING SIGNS OF A HEART ATTACK

Everyone should be aware of the warning signal of a heart attack. Shortness of breath, fatigue, nausea, and pain that radiates to the upper abdomen are the most common symptoms in women. The following are symptoms of a possible heart attack as described by the American Heart Association:

- Uncomfortable pressure, fullness, squeezing, or pain in the center of the chest that lasts more than a few minutes or goes away and comes back.
- Pain that spreads to the shoulders, neck, or arms.
- Chest discomfort with light-headedness, fainting, sweating, nausea, or shortness of breath.

Call 911 or your local emergency number if you think you are having a heart attack.

---

in life. Risk factors for atherosclerosis include a family history of heart disease, a diet high in fat and cholesterol, cigarette smoking, diabetes, obesity, and high blood pressure.

Hormones and Heart Disease

Doctors now know that there are multiple ways in which estrogen acts to protect women from heart disease. Estrogen lowers total blood cholesterol, increases the level of high density lipoproteins (HDL), the so-called good cholesterol that protects the heart, and decreases the level of low density lipoproteins (LDL), the so-called bad cholesterol that is harmful to the heart. Estrogen also has a direct beneficial effect on the blood vessels that lead to the heart, making the vessels dilate (widen), thereby increasing blood flow to the heart muscle. Estrogen also changes the lining of the blood vessels so that they are less likely to take up plaques (patches of fatty tissue on the inside lining of arteries) that can cause further narrowing.

Many studies have shown that current use of estrogen (as opposed to past use) offers the greatest protection against heart disease. Most experts believe that estrogen must be used long term as part of hormone replacement therapy (HRT) to provide the greatest benefits to the heart. Estrogen also protects women who have had previous heart disease from recurrence.

Another factor in the heart disease issue is progestin, a synthetic form of the female hormone progesterone. Progestin was added to HRT in the 1980s because it helps prevent cancer of the uterus. Women who were taking estrogen alone were shown to have an increased risk of developing an overgrowth of the endometrium (the lining of the uterus) that could eventually lead to cancer. Today, women who take HRT and who have not had a hysterectomy are advised to take both estrogen and progestin, so that the progestin can balance out the effects of the estrogen. Women who take both estrogen and progestin actually have a lower risk of endometrial cancer than women who do not take hormones. Progestin in high doses may counteract estrogen's beneficial effects on HDL and LDL, but in low doses, it may have a beneficial or neutral effect.

So what does all of this mean for you? Whether or not you have risk factors for heart disease, you should consider HRT and make an informed decision.

In addition to HRT, there are other steps you can take as a woman to protect yourself from heart disease. Knowing the risk factors for heart disease is the first step toward prevention.

Risk Factors for Heart Disease

Some risk factors for heart disease are not under your control. For example, you cannot change your age, your sex, or your heredity. But you can control most other risk factors. And you can take steps to reduce your risks. Heart disease is both preventable and treatable. A healthy lifestyle can be very effective in preventing heart disease. For best results, preventive efforts should begin early in life, long before potential health problems develop. The following are some well-known risk factors for heart disease.

Genetics. Heart disease runs in families. For example, if one or both of your parents had a heart attack before age 55, your risk of having a heart attack is increased. Be sure to discuss your family health history with your doctor so that he or she can provide advice on diet and lifestyle and perform any tests that may be needed.

Existing heart disease. If you have already had one heart attack, you are twice as likely to have another. Many people under age 50 who have had a heart attack show evidence of a problem with the heart or blood vessels that went undiagnosed and untreated. This underscores the importance of having routine checkups, especially if you have known risk factors for heart disease, such as family history.

High blood pressure. High blood pressure, or hypertension, occurs when higher than normal force is exerted by the blood against the walls of the arteries. Pressure in the arteries is created by the pumping of the heart. The arteries contract to help move the blood along. Each time the heart beats, pressure in the arteries increases; each time the heart relaxes between beats, the pressure drops. Thus, there are two pressures that are measured to evaluate the heart: an upper (systolic) pressure and a lower (diastolic) pressure.

As a general rule, a normal systolic pressure (the first number) is between 100 and 140, and a normal diastolic pressure is between 60 and 90. By taking several readings over a period of time, your doctor can work with you to determine what is a normal blood pressure for you.

Hypertension is a risk factor for heart disease and stroke. Having high blood pressure doubles your risk of a heart attack. This is true even in people who have mild hypertension. High blood pressure has no obvious symptoms. Left untreated, hypertension can also lead to kidney disease and vision loss. It is absolutely vital that you have your blood pressure checked regularly, especially if you are at high risk.

Women most at risk for high blood pressure include the following:

- Older women: more than half of all women over age 55 have hypertension
- Women in the last few months of pregnancy: this type of hypertension usually abates after the birth of the child
- Nonwhite women: African American women in particular are at risk

While hypertension cannot be cured, it responds well to a healthy lifestyle. Having regular checkups and taking your blood pressure medications as prescribed are vital. Also, good nutrition, exercise, weight control, a lifestyle free of cigarette smoking, and relaxation exercises may help to bring blood pressure down safely and effectively.

Cholesterol. A high level of cholesterol in the blood contributes to the development of plaque (patches of fatty tissue on the inside lining of arteries) in the coronary arteries and thus raises a woman's risk for heart disease. At normal levels, cholesterol is not harmful. In fact, the body needs it to function. Cholesterol lines the cells and helps carry out basic bodily functions. It insulates the nerves and allows normal transmission of nerve impulses. It contributes to the manufacture of certain hormones and vitamins, such as estrogen and vitamin D. The body is capable of manufacturing all of the cholesterol it needs.

It is easy to confuse cholesterol with fat, yet cholesterol is not a fat. It is a lipid—a waxy substance carried in the bloodstream along with several types of fat and protein. Fat and cholesterol are carried in the bloodstream by protein carriers called lipoproteins, so that they can travel easily through the blood to be deposited in the cells that require them to function normally. Depending on the type and amount, lipoproteins can either help prevent or contribute to heart disease. There are four types of lipoproteins, classified according to their weights: very low density (VLDL), low density (LDL, the "bad" cholesterol), high density (HDL, the "good" cholesterol), and very high density (VHDL).

The main carriers of cholesterol to the cells are the LDL, which leave fatty deposits called atheromas on the inside walls of the arteries, hampering the flow of blood and leading to atherosclerosis. Higher LDL levels in the blood reflect larger amounts of cholesterol in the bloodstream that can potentially clog the coronary arteries. The amount of LDL in your bloodstream is strongly influenced by the amount of fat and cholesterol in your diet. LDLs remain in the bloodstream longer in some people than in others; the more LDLs there are and the longer they remain in the bloodstream, the greater the risk to your health. One reason postmeno-pausal women are more susceptible to heart disease is that LDL levels tend to rise after menopause.

HDLs are considered the "good" carriers of cholesterol be-cause they move cholesterol out of the arteries and carry it to the liver, where it is excreted. In other words, HDLs act as scavengers of cholesterol. People with very low levels of HDL are more prone to heart attacks. Even when total cholesterol levels are relatively low, decreased HDL levels are associated with a greater incidence of heart attack.

The levels of HDL in the bloodstream are determined partly by genetic factors and partly by lifestyle factors, such as weight, level of physical activity, smoking, and diet. Before menopause, a woman's HDL level is generally higher than a man's. This may partly explain why women have a lower incidence of heart disease before menopause. On the basis of studies in men, it is thought that total cholesterol levels below 200 are desirable; total choles-terol levels above 240 are associated with increased risk of heart attack. Your cholesterol profile is incomplete, however, without measurements of HDL and LDL.

Because cholesterol plays a major role in heart disease, it is vital that you keep track of your blood cholesterol level. For an accurate assessment, you should be given a blood test to get your complete lipid profile, which includes your total cholesterol read-ing, the individual levels of HDL and LDL, and the ratio of HDL to total cholesterol. The ratio of HDL to total cholesterol is a better measure of your risk of heart disease than either total cholesterol or LDL levels. HDL levels of less than 35 may double your risk of heart attack. LDL levels should be less than 130; levels above 160 increase your heart attack risk further, particularly if you have other risk factors, such as obesity, a family history of heart disease, diabetes, or smoking. More significant than any of these individual numbers, however, is the ratio of total cholesterol to HDL. In general, a ratio of 4.5 or more indicates an increased risk for heart disease.

For information on how to control your blood cholesterol level, see Chapter 7.

Cigarette smoking. Smoking cigarettes increases a person's risk for heart disease at any age. Few young women have heart attacks, but those who do are much more likely to be smokers. Smoking affects the circulatory system (heart and blood vessels) in many ways.

The carbon monoxide contained in cigarette smoke reduces the blood's oxygen-carrying ability, so less oxygen is delivered to the heart and other organs. Smoking also decreases HDL cholesterol and raises LDL cholesterol. It damages the lining of the arteries, causing them to narrow and setting the stage for the development of plaque (patches of fatty tissue on the inside lining of arteries). Smoking also increases the likelihood of blood clot formation, irregular heart rhythms, and coronary spasms. And women who smoke reach menopause an average of 2 to 3 years earlier than nonsmokers; menopause itself is another risk factor for premature heart disease.

No matter how many years you have smoked, when you quit, your risk of heart disease declines. Within 2 years of stopping, your chances of a heart attack are cut in half; 10 years after stopping, your risk of heart attack will be about the same as if you had never smoked.

Diabetes. Diabetes doubles your risk of heart disease. Several studies suggest, however, that keeping your blood glucose (sugar) levels under strict control can significantly reduce this risk. Also, maintaining a normal weight is vital to controlling diabetes.

Excess weight. Being overweight significantly increases your risk of heart disease. But not all fat is created equal: women who tend to accumulate fat around the abdomen are at higher risk than those who collect fat in the hips and buttocks. Regardless of body shape, however, you are at lowest risk if you are at or below your ideal weight (see weight chart on page 121).

Sedentary lifestyle. Women who do not exercise are more likely to have a heart attack. Studies have shown that exercising as little as three times a week for 30 minutes each time will get your heart rate up to a level that increases its efficiency.

No matter what your age, an active lifestyle and a regular exercise program can keep your heart healthy. Exercise burns fat, thus helping to control your weight; it raises your protective HDL cholesterol levels and lowers your LDL cholesterol levels; it lowers your blood pressure and your baseline heart rate; and it promotes more efficient use of insulin, which helps prevent diabetes. It also increases your brain endorphin levels, to improve your sense of well-being, and helps you sleep better.

Stress. Studies have shown that people under a lot of stress may be at greater risk of heart disease. While the exact role stress plays in the development of heart disease remains unclear, it cannot be ruled out as a serious risk factor.

Popular stress relievers include regular exercise, yoga, meditation, massage, hobbies or crafts, plenty of sleep, and balancing your life to include both work and recreation. Choose the stress reliever that works best for you.

Age. The older you get, the higher your risk for heart disease. One in nine women between the ages of 45 and 64 has some form of cardiovascular disease; that ratio increases to one in three for women age 65 and older. Also, the older a woman is, the more likely she is to develop high blood pressure, high blood cholesterol levels, or diabetes. She is also more likely to become sedentary and overweight. All of these are major risk factors for heart disease.

Ethnicity. African American women are 25 percent more likely to die of heart disease than white women, and their death rate for stroke is 83 percent higher than that of white women. Hypertension is more common in African American women of all ages. They tend to develop it earlier in life and die from hypertension-related causes more frequently. Close attention to lifestyle factors that influence high blood pressure is vital for the health of black women.

Lowering Your Risk for Heart Disease

If you can make some simple lifestyle changes, you can significantly reduce your risk of heart disease. Here are just a few of the things you can do:

• **Stop smoking.** Ex-smokers lose their high-risk status within three years of quitting. When a woman stops smoking, her HDL cholesterol levels usually rise, improving her overall cholesterol profile.

• **Eat a healthful diet.** A low-fat diet that includes lots of whole grains, fruits, and vegetables will go a long way toward reducing your risk of heart disease. For more information about healthy eating in midlife, see Chapter 7.

• **Exercise.** Engage in aerobic activities, which increase your heart rate and use the large muscles of your body. Brisk walking, bicycling, and swimming are ideal for women in midlife. Exercises that place weight on the larger bones of your body, such as brisk walking, jogging, and stair climbing, are also good for keeping your bones strong and dense. Plan and discuss any exercise program with your doctor, particularly if you have not been physically active for a while. For more information about beginning an exercise program, see Chapter 7.

• **If you drink alcohol, do so in moderation.** Several studies have shown that moderate amounts of alcohol (one or two drinks per day) may help prevent heart disease, particularly among women. Alcohol appears to protect against heart disease by raising levels of HDL cholesterol (the "good" cholesterol). However, heavy drinking (more than three drinks per day) can damage the heart muscle, alter the heart's rhythm, and reduce blood flow from the heart. And three or four drinks per day can raise blood pressure and damage other vital organs such as the liver.

• **Control high blood pressure.** Have regular checkups, monitor your blood pressure, follow any recommended lifestyle changes (see Chapter 7), and take your medication as prescribed. Do not skip medications on days that you feel good.

• **Control your weight.** It is never too late to lose excess pounds through diet and exercise. See Chapter 7 for more information about maintaining a healthful weight.

• **Keep diabetes in check.** Work with your doctor and follow all recommendations about living with diabetes. This includes taking your medications as prescribed, checking your blood glucose (sugar), and maintaining a normal body weight.

• **Control stress.** There are a number of helpful techniques for controlling stress. Read Chapter 7 for tips on how to relieve your stress.

• **Consider hormone replacement therapy.** Talk to your doctor about the potential benefits of HRT and its protective effects on the heart.

STROKE

Stroke is a major cause of disability and death among women in their middle and later years, but it can often be prevented.

Most strokes occur when a blood clot or a small piece of atherosclerotic plaque blocks the flow of blood to the brain, interrupting the brain's supply of oxygen and nutrients. Stroke results in the sudden loss of brain function with possible paralysis, severe brain damage, or death.

Blockage of blood circulation to the brain may result from either cerebral thrombosis or cerebral embolism. Cerebral thrombosis occurs when a blood clot forms in one of the major blood vessels supplying the brain. It is most often associated with atherosclerosis in the brain or the neck. Factors that increase the risk of cerebral thrombosis from atherosclerosis are the same as those for heart disease in general: high blood pressure, diabetes, high blood levels of cholesterol, and cigarette smoking. Cerebral embolism involves a clot that forms in another part of the body, usually the heart or a major artery. The clot is then carried in the bloodstream until it lodges in a blood vessel that supplies the brain. This blocks the blood vessel, preventing it from delivering oxygen to that part of the brain, which then dies. Cerebral embolism is common in patients with heart disease and atherosclerosis of the large arteries.

Another major cause of stroke is cerebral hemorrhage, which

is bleeding into the brain tissue from a ruptured blood vessel. Cerebral hemorrhage can be caused by high blood pressure, abnormally formed arteries and veins, or, especially in older people, weakened walls of brain arteries.

Warning Signs of Stroke

Symptoms of stroke depend on the areas of the brain affected. The most common symptoms include sudden weakness, loss of sensation on one side of the body, partial or total loss of vision, dizziness, slurred speech, mental confusion, and headache. Symptoms often worsen over the next several hours or days as more brain tissue is affected. For this reason, a person who has had a stroke should see a doctor immediately. In some cases, the progression of symptoms leads to coma and death. In some minor strokes, a small clot in a brain artery may dislodge itself, allowing the brain tissue to recover. In these cases, symptoms disappear in less than a day.

Warning: Immediately call for emergency medical help if you experience any of the following warning signs of stroke:

- Sudden weakness or numbness of the face, arm, and leg on one side of the body
- Loss of speech or difficulty speaking or understanding speech
- Dimness or loss of vision
- Unexplained dizziness, unsteadiness, or sudden falls

Are You at Risk?

The best way to prevent stroke is to reduce your risk. Some risk factors for stroke are beyond your control. These include your age (the incidence of stroke more than doubles in each successive decade after age 55), your sex (women are 30 percent less likely to have a stroke than men), your ethnicity (stroke is more prevalent among African Americans), and whether you have a personal or family history of stroke. People with diabetes, particularly women, are more susceptible to stroke regardless of whether the diabetes is kept under control.

Women who are at risk for stroke are usually advised not to use oral contraceptives. The amount of estrogen in the birth control pill may increase the chances of blood clotting, which may lead to stroke. The low doses of estrogen in HRT, however, do not increase your risk of blood clots or stroke.

Other risk factors for stroke that are at least partly within your control include the following:

• **High blood pressure.** This is the most important risk factor for stroke. Because the risk of stroke rises as blood pressure rises, reducing blood pressure reduces the risk of stroke by putting less stress on the walls of the blood vessels in the brain. For this reason, it is vital that you have your blood pressure checked regularly and that you keep your blood pressure under control (see page 51). Take your blood pressure medication as prescribed, even if you feel fine. Avoid stress and do not smoke.

• **Heart disease.** People with heart disease have more than twice the risk of stroke than people who have healthy hearts. By taking steps to prevent heart disease you also lower your risk of stroke (see page 50). Follow a low-fat, low-cholesterol diet, maintain a healthy weight, and do not smoke.

• **Transient ischemic attacks.** Often, a major stroke is preceded by transient ischemic attacks, known also as TIAs. TIAs occur when a blood clot temporarily clogs an artery or an artery goes into spasm and part of the brain does not get the blood it needs. Symptoms include temporary weakness; clumsiness; loss of feeling in an arm, leg, or the side of the face; temporary loss of vision in one eye; temporary loss of speech or difficulty speaking; and sometimes dizziness, double vision, and staggering. The clot may dislodge itself, relieving the obstruction and allowing circulation to return to the affected brain tissue. As the tissue revives, symptoms gradually disappear. Unlike a stroke, when a TIA ends, there are no lasting effects. If you have any of these symptoms, consult your health-care provider without delay.

OSTEOPOROSIS

Osteoporosis, an often debilitating disease, causes bones to become thin, porous, and weak, so that they break easily. A combination of factors, including genetics, hormones, age, diet, and lifestyle, contribute to your chances of developing osteoporosis.

Osteoporosis affects 25 million Americans, mostly women. Along with heart disease and breast cancer, it is one of the three most serious diseases affecting women. Half of all women between ages 45 and 75 show beginning signs of osteoporosis. Research has shown that good nutrition and regular exercise can cut the numbers of women affected by this disease in half, perhaps even more.

Changing attitudes and improved technology have greatly altered the outlook for people with osteoporosis. Today, many women live 30 years or more after menopause. Improving the quality of those years by preventing the complications of osteoporosis has become an important goal for everyone. Although some bone loss is expected as people age, osteoporosis should no longer be viewed as an inevitable consequence of aging.

A Bit about Bones

Bone is living tissue that is continuously changing. A constant remodeling process is under way in response to the demands of the body. At certain times, calcium is taken out of the bones to replenish the calcium supply in the blood. If excessive, this process can cause the bone to become weaker, such as when your diet is too low in calcium and when you are sedentary. At other times, increased amounts of calcium enter the bones from the bloodstream, making them denser and stronger. This happens when a person does weight-bearing exercise regularly and eats a diet rich in calcium.

Calcium is a mineral that makes stronger bones and teeth and plays a significant role in muscle contraction, the function of the heart, the transmission of nerve impulses, and blood clotting. The body has many glandular systems that regulate and stabilize the calcium level in the blood. These systems are responsible for moving calcium in and out of bone and in and out of the bloodstream.

Estrogen plays a major role in preserving bone strength. When estrogen levels decline at menopause, bone dissolves more rapidly than it recalcifies (see graph). Therefore, more calcium is removed from bone than is replaced. These changes cause bone to become softer and more prone to fracture. Reversing this process is the primary step in preventing and treating osteoporosis.

Osteoporosis can be painful and crippling. After menopause, a woman's chances of fracturing a bone increase dramatically; just

DECREASING BONE STRENGTH AND DECLINING ESTROGEN LEVELS

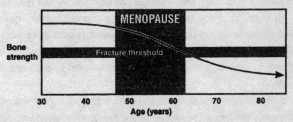

Effects of menopause on bone density

After about age 35, women gradually begin to lose bone strength and density. This process dramatically speeds up in the years after menopause, when estrogen production falls. A woman whose bone density is already low as she approaches menopause is at risk of fractures from bone loss unless she takes estrogen or other bone-building medications.

a minor fall or sudden twist may lead to a break. In their sixties, women may experience back pain as a result of the progressive loss of calcium in their vertebral bones; these "crush fractures" result in severe compression of the bones of the spine. Susceptible women may also fracture their wrist after a fall. The most significant bone problem occurs typically after age 70, when fracture of the head of the thigh bone, or femur, may take place. This is commonly referred to as fracture of the hip. Those who recover can be permanently limited in their ability to walk without pain. Hip fractures may result in immobilization, hospitalization, and dependence. Hip fractures can also be associated with long-term disability and an accelerated death rate from complications during surgery and from immobilization.

The physical deformities caused by osteoporosis are obvious in some women. An older woman with advanced osteoporosis loses height, is hunched over, has a protruding abdomen, and often walks with an unsteady gait. This is because as the bones of the spine lose density, the vertebrae collapse, forcing the rib cage to tilt downward toward the pelvis. A curvature in the upper spine creates a second curve in the lower spine, pushing the internal organs outward. Because of the compression in the spinal column, a woman with osteoporosis can lose up to 8 inches in height.

A woman's appearance and self-esteem may change when osteoporosis reaches an advanced stage. Along with being uncomfortable and perhaps disabled, she may find that clothing does not fit properly, and she may feel awkward. Activities of daily living, such as shopping or attending religious services, may become more difficult. Limited mobility results in feelings of dependence and isolation.

Diagnosing Osteoporosis

Special X-ray techniques designed to screen women at the time of menopause are used to detect osteoporosis. Such screening helps identify early signs of osteoporosis before fractures occur. Tests such as dual energy X-ray absorptiometry (DEXA) or dual photon absorptiometry (DPA) can measure the density of the bones of the vertebrae of the lower back and hip.

A bone-screening test of the spine or hip compares your bone density to that of other women of your age and women of age 35—the age when bone density begins to decrease. Women with comparatively low bone density are more likely to have fractures later in life. If you have a bone-screening test around the time of menopause and again a year later, the readings can help you and your doctor set a baseline measurement for evaluating your rate of bone loss and help monitor the effectiveness of treatment.

Special urine and blood tests can predict bone loss after menopause. These tests measure the amounts of calcium and other by-products of bone breakdown in urine or blood and are useful in determining whether a woman is at risk for osteoporosis.

Who Is at Risk?

There are several risk factors for osteoporosis. Some are within your control, others are not.

Sex. Women have an acceleration of bone loss immediately after reaching menopause, whether it is natural or surgical menopause. This is why it is important to begin HRT as soon as menopause is diagnosed, before significant bone loss has occurred.

Genetics. If your mother, aunt, or sister had fractures caused by osteoporosis, you are also at risk. A genetic marker for osteoporosis, related to the vitamin D receptor in cells, has been located.

Body size. Small-boned, thin women have a dramatically greater risk of osteoporosis than heavy, more muscular women. Bones respond to a higher weight load by forming new bone tissue to meet the demand: the heavier you are, the greater the stress on your body, and the more bone is formed. More weight means more gravitational pull on the body and more work for the bones and muscles—all of which helps to keep the bones strong. More body fat means more estrogen production within the body, which helps prevent osteoporosis. However, this does not justify being overweight, which carries health risks that are far greater than this one benefit. Weight-bearing exercise can provide similar benefits.

Skin color. The fairer your complexion, the greater your risk of osteoporosis. White women, followed by Asian women, are at the highest risk for osteoporosis. Hispanic women from Central America have a lower risk of fractures. African American women develop osteoporosis less often, perhaps because of heavier bones or favorable hormonal differences. However, recent studies show that African American women who have other risk factors for osteoporosis, such as corticosteroid use, surgical menopause, and lactose intolerance, are at increased risk for hip fracture.

Other medical conditions. Medical problems may make you more vulnerable to bone loss. Diabetes, kidney or liver diseases, celiac disease, Crohn's disease, hyperthyroidism, hypothyroidism, hyperparathyroidism, and gastrointestinal surgery are some medical conditions that interfere with the body's absorption and use of calcium and other important nutrients necessary for building and maintaining strong bones.

Bone formation is a complex process involving interaction of organs, hormones, and minerals. Any defect or disease that affects metabolism, the endocrine system, the liver, or kidney function or any illness that requires extended immobilization causes calcium loss, which leads to bone loss.

Medications. Several medications interfere with how your body absorbs calcium. Some drugs that affect calcium balance include corticosteroids, anticonvulsants, antacids containing aluminum, and diuretics. Ask your doctor if prescription drugs and over-the-counter drugs that you use affect how your body absorbs and uses calcium—and what you should do to compensate for this.

Diet. Calcium intake is a vital part of preventing osteoporosis. A low-calcium diet contributes to osteoporosis. Many young women today do not get enough calcium in their diet. Because peak bone mass is reached by age 18 to 20, it is especially important to get adequate calcium early in life. However, calcium remains important throughout the life span, regardless of a woman's age.

If you have eaten plenty of foods high in calcium throughout your life and you have exercised regularly, you can expect to reach menopause with strong, healthy bones. But if you have not gotten enough calcium in the past, it is never too late to start. Taking in the recommended amounts of calcium each day at menopause and after may help keep your bones strong. For more information about calcium, see Chapter 7.

However, a high-calcium diet alone will not protect against the loss of bone that naturally results from declining levels of estrogen. Because most women get only about 500 milligrams of calcium per day from their diet, many doctors recommend taking calcium supplements to bring the total amount up to the recommended level (1,000 to 1,500 milligrams per day for most women). Ask your doctor to recommend an appropriate calcium supplement for you.

Vitamin D in the body allows absorption of calcium. Vitamin D is formed on bare skin when a person is outdoors in the sun. It is stored in the liver until needed and then converted in the kidneys to its active form. However, many people do not get enough sunlight because of clothing, long periods spent indoors, long and dark winters, or smog. Others avoid sun exposure because they are concerned about skin cancer or rapid aging of the skin. For these reasons, vitamin D has been added to many commercially prepared dairy products.

Fat also affects calcium absorption. If fat consumption is too high or too low, calcium absorption is depressed. Calcium requires the presence of some fat for absorption, so do not try to eliminate all fat from your diet, even when you are trying to lose weight. The preferred forms of fat are those found in whole natural foods, such as raw seeds and nuts, vegetable oils, and fish. The fats to avoid are saturated fats found in foods such as red meat, high-fat dairy products, shortening, processed foods, and some vegetable oils, such as coconut and palm oil. Keeping fat-calorie intake to between 25 percent and 30 percent of total calories is generally a good idea.

Another dietary factor in osteoporosis is protein. High levels of protein may stimulate the breakdown of bone and encourage long-term bone loss. (A very high protein diet is one that contains twice the body's daily need for protein.) This is because the end products of digestion of protein-rich foods are acids, such as sulfuric acid, which the body eliminates in the urine. In response, the kidneys eliminate calcium to balance this acid. Even a young person who eats too much protein may lose significant amounts of calcium. Postmenopausal women who are not taking HRT are at greater risk from this dietary cause of calcium loss.

A diet high in salt is also a contributing factor to osteoporosis. It has long been known that too much salt can lead to high blood pressure (a major risk factor for heart disease) in people who are "salt sensitive." Salt also causes the kidneys to excrete more calcium in the urine. Over the long run, this loss of calcium can contribute to osteoporosis.

Drinking and smoking. Alcohol and cigarettes both contribute to a woman's risk of osteoporosis.

Heavy alcohol intake has been linked to inadequate absorption of calcium. It also puts stress on the liver, interfering with the body's utilization of vitamin D. Heavy use of alcohol also leads to accidents, falls, and fractures. Many hip fractures in older women are caused by falls related to the use of alcohol.

Women who smoke lose bone faster than nonsmokers. Smokers generally experience menopause earlier than nonsmokers, and the premature drop in estrogen caused by early menopause may be responsible for diminished depositing of calcium into the bones. Smokers reach menopause with bones that are already weaker than those of nonsmokers. Studies have shown higher rates of bone fractures in postmenopausal smokers, probably because smoking inhibits estrogen production by the ovaries. Because smokers tend to weigh less and exercise less than nonsmokers, their risk of osteoporosis is even higher. Smokers who are also thin are at highest risk.

Physical activity. Lack of exercise can lead to osteoporosis. When people are inactive, their bones lose calcium. Conversely, when a person exercises regularly, the bones become stronger. Weight-bearing exercises, such as jogging, brisk walking, or stair climbing, are best. There is no question that osteoporosis is related to a sedentary lifestyle.

If you have any combination of these symptoms, talk to your doctor. He or she will examine you and perform tests to determine whether you have osteoporosis.

WARNING SIGNS OF OSTEOPOROSIS

The following are warning signs of osteoporosis:

- Chronic low back pain
- Loss of height
- Leg cramps at night
- Joint pain
- Tooth loss
- Periodontal (gum) disease

Preventing Osteoporosis

Exercise helps to build and maintain strong bones. Like muscle, bone grows stronger with use. Bone density depends directly on how much the bone is used. The more they are used, the more calcium is deposited in the bones and the stronger the bones become.

You do not have to be an athlete to benefit from exercise. Muscle-strengthening exercises help reverse the decline in muscle mass and muscle strength that comes with aging, and they may also help increase bone density. But the best type of exercise for building strong bones is weight-bearing exercise, such as jogging, skipping rope, brisk walking, stair climbing, or dancing. To benefit fully, exercise for about 30 minutes at a pace fast enough to get your heart pumping a bit faster than normal. If you have arthritis or other joint problems, ask your doctor which type of exercise is best for you. Even activities such as gardening and housework can help maintain bone strength. The more you exercise, the greater the health benefits will be.

It is never too late to start exercising. If you are not physically active, start an exercise program as soon as possible. However, talk to your doctor first about which type of exercise is best for you if you are currently inactive. For more information about starting an exercise program, see Chapter 7.

Prevention is the best way to avoid the bone fractures, severe discomfort, and permanent disfigurement of osteoporosis. Once detected, osteoporosis can be controlled to a certain degree, so it is a good idea to begin preventive measures now. Determine your risk factors for osteoporosis, then take steps to deal with those factors that are within your control. Regular, weight-bearing exercise will make your bones stronger and less susceptible to fracture. A diet high in calcium with adequate levels of vitamin D and other bone-protecting substances is essential for all women—no matter what age. For more information about combating osteoporosis through diet and exercise, see Chapter 7.

Hormone-Replacement Therapy and Osteoporosis

Estrogen is important to the health of your bones. This female hormone improves calcium absorption and reduces the amount of calcium eliminated in the urine. Taking estrogen as part of HRT is the best way to protect your bones. If you are at high risk for osteoporosis or you have already begun to lose bone mass, the answer to whether you should take estrogen may well be yes.

Not all women are candidates for HRT. Women with estrogen-related cancers, such as breast cancer, are advised not to take HRT. Other women may find HRT undesirable because of its side effects. And some women are not comfortable with the idea of taking hormones and drugs to control a natural life process. Even though HRT appears to be protective against bone loss and heart disease, the long-term effects, such as the possible risk of uterine and breast cancer, cause many women to say no to HRT.

There are alternative ways to get protection. A number of drugs are now available that may help. These include calcitonin and alendronate, both of which are discussed in Chapter 6. For more information about HRT and osteoporosis, see Chapter 5. For more information about decreasing your risk of osteoporosis, see Chapter 7.

OSTEOARTHRITIS

Osteoarthritis is the most common form of arthritis and appears most often in the later years of life. It is a degenerative disease related to the wear and tear of aging and involves deterioration of the joint cartilage at the ends of the bones. Osteoarthritis is often a mild condition, causing no symptoms in many and only occasional joint pain and stiffness in others. Still, some women may experience considerable pain and disability.

The onset of osteoarthritis can be subtle, beginning with morning joint stiffness. As the disease progresses, there is pain when you move the joint. The pain worsens with prolonged motion and is relieved by resting the joint.

Though most older people have some degree of osteoarthritis, the condition can occur at any age, especially after a joint injury. The joints most likely to be affected are those of the feet, toes, and fingers and the joints of the weight-bearing bones, such as the knees, hips, ankles, and spine.

Many menopausal women complain of aching joints. Whether

it is age or hormones, body aches and pains after menopause seem to appear in women who have not experienced them before or intensify in women who have. Osteoarthritis has many causes, including injury and complications from some diseases. A tendency toward developing osteoarthritis may also be hereditary.

Your doctor can diagnose osteoarthritis based on your history of joint pain and on symptoms of joint tenderness, swelling, and pain when you move the joint. An X-ray examination of the joints involved can confirm cartilage loss.

As yet, there is no cure for osteoarthritis. Symptoms may be relieved by painkillers and nonsteroidal anti-inflammatory drugs (NSAIDs), which reduce joint swelling. Physical therapy, including exercises and heat treatment, can often relieve symptoms. Probably the best thing you can do to relieve the pain, stiffness, and swelling caused by osteoarthritis is to maintain a healthful body weight (see page 121). Carrying excess weight increases stress on the weight-bearing joints, which, in turn, increases pain and discomfort. Weight control alone can greatly ease any discomfort and stiffness you experience.

BREAST CANCER

Research has not determined whether the drop in estrogen associated with menopause affects a woman's risk of developing breast cancer.

Surgical removal of the ovaries, which causes artificial menopause and stops a woman's natural production of estrogen, significantly reduces her risk of developing breast cancer, especially if she is in her midthirties.

RISK OF DEVELOPING BREAST CANCER BY AGE

AGE	RISK
25	1 in 19,608
30	1 in 2,525
35	1 in 622
40	1 in 217
45	1 in 93
50	1 in 50
55	1 in 33
60	1 in 24
65	1 in 17
70	1 in 14
75	1 in 11
80	1 in 10
85	1 in 9
90	1 in 8
95	1 in 8

The size and shape of the breasts are altered when estrogen levels fall after menopause. The alveoli, the tiny sacs where breast milk is made and stored, begin to disappear, and the milk ducts decrease in number. But because hormones and aging play a role in the development of many kinds of breast cancer, it is difficult to determine the specific impact menopause-related changes have on a woman's risk of developing the disease. Although it would seem that the risk of developing estrogen-dependent cancers of the breast would be reduced after menopause, statistics show that the number of estrogen-dependent cancers increases steadily until ages 60 to 74—about 10 to 15 years after estrogen levels fall at menopause. And for reasons that are not yet clear, breast cancer is far more prevalent in women over age 50. In fact, the older you are, the greater your chances of developing breast cancer. The disease rarely occurs before age 20, and the chances of developing breast cancer gradually increase after that, leveling off somewhat after menopause, then rising again at age 65.

But there are many things you can do to protect yourself against breast cancer. The first is to determine your risk factors. A family history definitely plays a significant role. If your mother, sister, or both have had breast cancer, your risk is 2 to 10 times higher than that of a woman whose nearest female relatives are free of the disease. Also, the longer a woman continues to have natural menstrual cycles, the greater her chances of developing breast cancer. Women who have their first baby after age 35 are twice as likely to develop breast cancer, as are those who give birth while in their teens. Breast cancer also occurs more frequently among overweight women and those who have previously had cancer of the other breast, ovary, or uterus. Your chances of developing breast cancer probably increase with each additional risk factor you have.

If you have even one risk factor for breast cancer, you should have regular breast examinations every 3 to 6 months. In addition, all women should perform monthly breast self-examination and have their doctor perform a breast examination once a year, beginning at age 20. The current recommendation is for women to have a baseline mammogram at age 40 and then to have a regular mammogram every 1 or 2 years until 50, when they should begin having mammograms every year. The frequency at which your doctor will recommend you have mammograms before 50 will depend on your risk of developing breast cancer.

ALZHEIMER'S DISEASE

Estrogen plays a role in brain function, especially memory, and declining estrogen levels after menopause may be linked to Alzheimer's disease, as well as other types of dementia. However, these findings are preliminary; women should not feel that once they reach menopause they automatically have an increased likelihood of developing Alzheimer's disease. It is important to note that researchers have linked Alzheimer's disease to genetic inheritance, so declining estrogen levels are not likely to be the only factor causing the disease.

Estrogen promotes the growth of brain cells, specifically in the regions of the cerebral cortex and the hypothalamus. Researchers have discovered that estrogen also prompts the growth of nerve cell extensions and supports the communication links between nerve cells in the brain.

In Alzheimer's disease, nerve-cell changes in certain regions of the brain result in the death of a large number of those cells. Symptoms begin slowly and become steadily worse. In the early stages of the disease, people forget very recent events but can clearly recall events that took place many years earlier. Later, people with Alzheimer's disease can no longer remember events of the distant past, and they may not be able to recognize friends and family members. Judgment and the ability to reason also decline as the disease progresses. Fatigue and anxiety worsen the mental disabilities and make it more difficult for the person to cope with daily life. Eventually, people with Alzheimer's disease cannot care for themselves, and most become bedridden. In their weakened condition, they are vulnerable to pneumonia and other infectious diseases. Most die from such diseases 8 to 10 years after developing Alzheimer's disease.

Fifty percent of Americans over age 85 have Alzheimer's disease, and the majority are women. One reason for this is that women generally live longer than men, and Alzheimer's is a disease that generally affects older people. Women might develop Alzheimer's disease more readily because they lose estrogen at menopause. This theory has been supported by the findings in several recent studies in which women on HRT were less likely to have Alzheimer's disease than those who had not taken estrogen. Higher estrogen doses were also associated with a lower risk for the disease.

5

Hormone Replacement Therapy

This chapter is an in-depth discussion of hormone replacement therapy (HRT), the often debated treatment for the symptoms of menopause.

WHAT IS HORMONE REPLACEMENT THERAPY?

Here is a quick review of the female hormones and the roles they play. Estrogen and progesterone control the female reproductive system. They also have an effect on many other systems and tissues in your body. These hormones play a role in blood cholesterol levels and the health of the heart, in building bones and other aspects of growth, in the health of the skin and hair, and in behavior and brain function. As hormone production declines at menopause, bones begin to thin, quite rapidly for the first 5 to 10 years after menopause. As time passes, women lose their natural resistance to heart disease; by age 65, the risk of heart attack is as great in women as it is in men.

HRT is a medical treatment with prescription drugs in which a woman's declining hormone levels are restored to premenopausal levels. Doctors advise women to take HRT to treat symptoms of menopause such as hot flashes and vaginal dryness on a long-term basis to help reduce their chances of developing osteoporosis and heart disease.

The use of HRT is not new. Doctors have been prescribing hormones for many years, and estrogen and progesterone are the most extensively studied hormones in the history of medicine.

THE HISTORY OF HORMONE REPLACEMENT THERAPY

Estrogen has been used to treat the symptoms of menopause for years. In the 1950s and 1960s, doctors readily prescribed estrogen to relieve menopausal symptoms. By 1975, estrogen was one of the top prescription drugs in the US.

Then in the mid-1970s, medical studies reported that for postmenopausal women who used estrogen therapy alone, risk of developing endometrial cancer, which affects the lining of the uterus, was increased 10-fold. Researchers soon discovered that adding progestin, a synthetic form of the female hormone progesterone, to estrogen therapy not only protected women from this cancer but also resulted in a lower incidence of endometrial cancer than found in women who took no hormones at all. So progestin was added to the hormone replacement regimen for women who still had their uterus. This became the treatment that is now called HRT.

Further research revealed more about estrogen's positive effects on heart disease and osteoporosis. As a result, HRT has gained more popularity among doctors and the women they treat.

The Hormone Replacement Therapy Controversy

Today, doctors prescribe relatively lower doses of estrogen and progesterone. The commonly used doses are actually less than what a woman's body produces naturally before menopause. How much estrogen to prescribe, with or without progestin and in what form, is determined on an individual basis, depending on each woman's symptoms and health history. HRT is prescribed on a long-term basis to help protect against heart disease, osteoporosis, and other aging-related conditions, such as Alzheimer's disease and colon cancer.

On one side of the HRT debate are those who view menopause as a condition to be treated. Noting the many health problems related to the lack of estrogen, these proponents of HRT encourage women to replace their body's estrogen for the rest of their lives. They support HRT not only as a treatment for symptoms of menopause but also as a long-term preventive measure against aging-related diseases. Evidence is mounting that, for many women, the hormonal changes at menopause do contribute to chronic diseases and early death. In fact, recent studies have shown that women on HRT live 3 years longer than women not on HRT.

Those on the other side of the HRT debate criticize what they term the "medicalization" of a natural life process. They disagree with the view that the changes at midlife are like a disease that requires medication. They question whether HRT should be prescribed as a long-term preventive treatment before there are enough long-term studies to guarantee its safety and effectiveness. In addition, some object to the routine prescribing of hormones for healthy women because of the risks that are known to be associated with the use of hormones.

The views of many women and doctors fall somewhere in-between these two opposing opinions. These people feel that each case should be decided individually. A woman's risk for heart disease, osteoporosis, breast cancer, and other health problems and her personal feelings about taking hormones must be considered.

The use of replacement hormones after menopause has overwhelming benefits for most women. As life expectancy has increased over the years, more and more women live a significant portion of their lives after menopause. The risk of heart disease and osteoporosis increases as a woman ages. Estrogens can help to significantly decrease the risk of both conditions. HRT has both benefits and risks, some of which scientists know a little about, but others that have yet to be determined. Only many years of careful study can provide the answers.

If you decide to take hormones either to relieve the symptoms you have today or to prevent the possibility of disease in the future, it is important that you carefully explore your options. Your decision should take into account your health, your lifestyle, and the reasons you are taking these drugs.

HOW HORMONE REPLACEMENT THERAPY WORKS

It is very difficult to understand how hormones work, because we do not really know everything about them. It is known that in order to work, a hormone needs a receptor site to get into a cell. Once in the cell, the hormone triggers a series of reactions within the body.

Many drugs are used to mimic the effects of hormones. Researchers once thought that every drug that fit a given receptor site would cause the same effect. But further investigation has shown that some drugs seem to fit a receptor site without causing an effect. Instead, they simply attach to the receptor site so that a hormone cannot use the receptor site and do its work. These drugs are called hormone blockers. Tamoxifen, which is used to treat breast cancer, is a hormone blocker.

However, not all receptor sites are the same in every cell. The receptor sites in the uterus, for example, are completely different from those in the breast, so progestin may change estrogen's effects in the uterus but imitate its actions in the breast. This may help to explain why progestin, when taken as part of HRT, helps fight uterine cancer but does not have the same effect on breast cancer. In the breast, progestin may instead stimulate estrogen.

Researchers are just beginning to understand how hormones and HRT work. And as the investigation continues, they are hoping to discover the ideal hormone: one that will protect the uterus and the breasts from cancer, relieve menopausal symptoms, and prevent osteoporosis and heart disease.

FORMS OF HORMONE REPLACEMENT THERAPY

The most common hormones used in HRT are forms of estrogen, progesterone, and sometimes testosterone. HRT comes in a variety of forms, or delivery methods. It can be taken by mouth, through the skin, or through the vagina. Each form has its advantages and drawbacks.

Oral preparations—tablets taken by mouth—reach the bloodstream by way of the digestive system and must pass through the liver. Estrogen, progestin, and testosterone can all be taken orally. Estrogen is also available as a transdermal skin patch and as such is not swallowed or ingested and therefore avoids the digestive system and the liver. Whether the hormones travel through the digestive system may make a difference in their effects on your body and ultimately on your symptoms.

Other nonoral forms of estrogen include injections, vaginal rings, and vaginal creams. While not yet available in the US, subcutaneous (under the skin) pellets and estrogen gel may one day be additional options. Nonoral progestins include injections, intrauterine devices, and vaginal suppositories. The future of progestins may include transdermal progestins and vaginal progesterone gel. Testosterone is available in tablet form or as a cream.

You may choose just one form of HRT—taking all hormones in tablet form, for example. Tablets are the most common form prescribed. Or you may try a combination of forms. If you have your uterus, your health-care provider might prescribe an estrogen patch with oral progestin tablets, for example.

Oral Estrogens

Pills are the most common form of HRT prescribed today. An advantage to taking oral estrogen is that its effect on the liver's regulation of cholesterol has a well-known association with a marked increase in high density lipoprotein (HDL, or "good") cholesterol and decrease in low density lipoprotein (LDL, or "bad") cholesterol. Nonoral estrogen, which does not pass through the liver, also raises HDL cholesterol, but it may take a longer time to do so. Estrogen, whether taken orally or by skin patch, provides cardiovascular protection, and estrogen's effect on HDL cholesterol is only one of the ways it does so. Estrogen also has other beneficial effects on the heart, including a direct effect on the coronary arteries, which supply oxygen to the heart muscle, to stay open and take up less plaque (fatty tissue on the inside lining of arteries).

Some women report severe heartburn when they take tablets of any kind. These women may prefer to take estrogen in the form of the skin patch, which provides the same benefit.

Transdermal Estrogens

The second most common HRT delivery method is the skin patch. The patch sticks to the skin and releases a steady flow of hormones directly into the bloodstream. A new patch is applied once or twice a week, to the upper arm, buttocks, or abdomen. A small percentage of women may develop minor skin irritation from its use.

In most cases, the patch is as efficient as an oral tablet in delivering estrogen to the body and in treating menopausal symptoms such as hot flashes and vaginal dryness. This method also appears to be as effective as oral estrogen in limiting the accelerated period of bone loss that occurs after menopause and in preventing osteoporosis. The patch also has a positive effect on increasing HDL and lowering LDL cholesterol levels.

For many women, an advantage to the patch is that it is easier to use than taking pills every day, since the patch needs to be changed only once or twice a week.

Estrogen Vaginal Creams

Estrogen vaginal creams are often used by women who want relief from the vaginal symptoms of menopause, such as vaginal dryness or painful intercourse. These creams, inserted by a woman directly into her vagina two or more times a week, are one of the best ways to treat urinary or vaginal symptoms of menopause. They produce a high local concentration of estrogen, which is what makes these creams particularly helpful in treating these symptoms.

Depending on the dose prescribed, some estrogen from these creams may be absorbed into the bloodstream. For this reason, if you regularly use estrogen vaginal creams, you are advised to also take progestin in order to reduce the risk of endometrial cancer.

Applying the cream just before bedtime reduces vaginal leakage and allows more time for absorption. These creams are not meant to be used as a lubricant for intercourse, however, and do not work for this purpose.

Oral Progestin

Progestin must be taken in conjunction with estrogen to help reduce the risk of endometrial cancer that occurs when estrogen is taken alone. Taking progestin along with estrogen for several days per month limits the growth of uterine lining, preventing excessive buildup and thus minimizing the risk of cancer. Currently, progestin is prescribed most often in tablet form.

Testosterone

Occasionally, testosterone is added to the HRT regimen, usually in women who report a decreased libido. Women who have not had a hysterectomy still need to take progestin to reduce their risk of endometrial cancer.

HOW HORMONE REPLACEMENT THERAPY IS ADMINISTERED

There is no single HRT regimen. Which days of the month you take hormones and which hormones you take—estrogen alone or combined with progestin and/or testosterone—make up your HRT regimen. Regimens vary from woman to woman, depending on the type and severity of symptoms and individual health history. Unless you have had a hysterectomy, you are typically prescribed a combined regimen of estrogen and progestin.

You may need to try a few regimens before finding the one that works best for you. Fitting the right dose and hormone type with the right administration route and the right schedule can take adjustments and time. Be patient and flexible. Then you will be able to determine which regimen is most manageable and convenient for you and your lifestyle.

Combined Estrogen–Progestin Therapy

For women who have their uterus, the two most commonly used medication schedules are continuous combined or cyclic therapy. Both have advantages and disadvantages.

One widely used HRT schedule—cyclic therapy—tries to mimic the premenopausal ovarian hormone cycle. The most common timetable using this regimen involves taking a daily dose of estrogen, with a daily dose of progestin added for the first 12 to 14 days of the month.

Some women report side effects such as breast tenderness or fluid retention. In addition, most women on a cyclic regimen experience withdrawal bleeding when the progestin is stopped. Withdrawal bleeding is generally less heavy than regular menstrual bleeding and is accompanied by fewer cramps. (Sometimes withdrawal bleeding does not occur at all, which is not a cause for concern. However, if bleeding occurs at any time other than when expected, it should be reported to your doctor, because it could signal a problem.) Lowering the dose of progestin usually alleviates the side effects, but progestin should not be eliminated altogether in women who still have a uterus.

A popular alternative to cyclic therapy is continuous combined therapy, which calls for both estrogen and progestin every day of the month, 365 days a year. This regimen commonly uses lower doses of progestin because it is taken more often. Many women still experience some irregular bleeding for the first 6 months of therapy. Although the bleeding usually subsides over time, some women have difficulty dealing with its irregularity. A switch to the cyclic regimen, in which this bleeding occurs predictably each month, may be preferable.

In all forms of combined therapy, testosterone may be included. It is generally combined with estrogen in tablet form.

Estrogen Alone

Also called unopposed estrogen, the estrogen regimen involves taking only estrogen with no added progestin. This regimen is generally recommended for women who have had their uterus removed or for those who cannot tolerate even low doses of progestin. If you use this method and still have your uterus, you are advised to have an annual endometrial biopsy (removal of cells from the lining of the uterus for microscopic examination) to check for cancer.

Making a Choice

When faced with the decision of which method or regimen of HRT is best for you, be sure to discuss fully with your doctor which is the most effective method for your particular needs. You should also consider which method is most convenient for you and your lifestyle. Too often, women stop taking HRT because the method they choose becomes bothersome. Keep in mind that if one method becomes problematic, your doctor can recommend another option. But make sure that you give each method that you try an opportunity to work. Try one method for at least 3 months before switching to another, unless, of course, the symptoms are unbearable or make you uneasy. Working together, you and your doctor should be able to find the method that works best for you.

THE BENEFITS OF HORMONE REPLACEMENT THERAPY

Most doctors agree that the benefits of HRT outweigh the risks for most women. Research continues to support the positive role of long-term therapy in the prevention of life-threatening diseases, such as osteoporosis and heart disease. The known benefits of HRT are explained below.

Preventing Heart Disease

Heart disease is the major cause of death in women over age 65. When postmenopausal women who take estrogen are compared to those who do not, the estrogen users are found to have about a 50 percent reduction in risk of fatal heart attack. This lower risk has been seen in all groups of women, even those with risk factors for heart disease, such as high blood pressure, high cholesterol levels, obesity, smoking, or a family history of early heart attack. It is thought that estrogen offers these benefits in several ways—by lowering total cholesterol levels and by enhancing the ability of coronary blood vessels to dilate, permitting more blood flow to the heart and other vital organs.

In 1991, the National Institutes of Health (NIH) began the Postmenopausal Estrogen/Progestin Interventions (PEPI) trial to study the effects of HRT on risk factors for heart disease in postmenopausal women. This 3-year study supported the results of many other medical trials that had shown that HRT produces significant elevations in HDL ("good") cholesterol, thus reducing a woman's risk for heart disease. The study included nearly 900 women who were randomly assigned to one of five treatment groups, including a placebo (no treatment) group and various combinations of estrogen, progestin, and natural progesterone therapy. All hormone regimens produced significantly greater increases in HDL cholesterol than did the placebo, with estrogen alone having the most positive effect. The PEPI study also showed that all of the hormone regimens produced significant decreases in LDL ("bad") cholesterol, offering even more protection against heart disease. While high doses of progestins that are prescribed along with estrogen to prevent endometrial cancer may reduce some of the favorable effects of estrogen on the heart, there is still a substantial gain of protection compared to women who do not take estrogen at all.

While the findings of the PEPI study are encouraging, 3 years was not enough time to see if HRT actually reduced the incidence of heart disease among the women in the study. A longer study, the Women's Health Initiative, began in 1993, and will follow women for 9 to 12 years to measure the effects of hormones on the rate of heart disease. This study will be able to provide more insight into HRT's effect on the heart. In addition, while HRT appears to help prevent heart disease, other variables may be involved in lowering heart disease risk. Women who take estrogen therapy tend to be healthier and more affluent and therefore already at a lower risk of heart disease. Better diet and health care among women on HRT also may contribute to the lower death rate.

All women need to understand the beneficial effects of HRT

on the prevention of heart disease. If you have risk factors for heart disease, talk to your doctor. Even if you do not have risk factors for heart disease, you will benefit from estrogen for long-term heart disease protection.

Preventing Osteoporosis

A lot of research has demonstrated that replacing estrogen effectively stops the bone loss associated with menopause and reduces a woman's risk for fracture, even when treatment is not begun until well after menopause. The best HRT-related protection against osteoporosis, however, occurs when HRT is begun within 3 years of menopause and is continued for 10 years or more. Estrogen must be taken over a long term in order for its effects on bone to be realized. The hormone's therapeutic effects wear off soon after therapy is discontinued. In fact, when estrogen is stopped, bone density can decrease as rapidly as it does in a woman just entering menopause who has not begun any sort of treatment.

Contrary to popular belief, HRT can still have positive effects even if a women already has osteoporosis. Estrogen is approved by the US Food and Drug Administration (USFDA) for treatment of osteoporosis. It is never too late to begin therapy to avoid bone loss. Even when begun in a woman's seventies or eighties, HRT can still inhibit further bone loss to a significant degree. The effects of HRT on the prevention of bone fracture is another area under study by the Women's Health Initiative.

Women who take hormones must realize, however, that HRT cannot *reverse* bone loss. Osteoporosis cannot be cured. Instead, hormones primarily slow bone loss, thus preserving existing bone. And because no treatment significantly stimulates bone growth, all women—including those on HRT—are encouraged to maintain healthy bones by eating right, exercising regularly, engaging in other habits of healthy living, and avoiding situations in which they might fall and fracture a bone (for example, wearing spike heels, climbing ladders, or slipping on loose rugs).

Preventing Colon Cancer

Studies have shown a significant decrease in colon cancer and deaths related to it among women using HRT. Because colon cancer is a major problem for older women—it is the second most common cancer in women, after breast cancer—this may turn out to be an important benefit of hormone use.

A high-fiber, low-fat diet, rich in vegetables and fruits, can also help to prevent colon cancer. Calcium, vitamin D, and exercise may also help reduce this risk.

Relief of Menopausal Symptoms

Short-term HRT can reduce or eliminate many of the uncomfortable physical symptoms of menopause. Here is a description of how HRT helps specific symptoms.

• **Hot flashes.** For most women, HRT decreases the occurrence of hot flashes. Estrogen is widely considered the most effective form of therapy for this uncomfortable symptom of menopause. To treat hot flashes, your goal should be to find the lowest dose that will prevent discomfort. You and your doctor can work together to achieve this goal. A good way to begin is to keep a diary of your hot flashes. Your doctor will probably start with the average therapeutic dose and adjust it down or up depending on side effects.

One or two weeks after starting HRT, you will find that hot flashes begin to subside significantly. If you stop taking estrogen, however, your hot flashes may return.

For hot flashes that occur during perimenopause, many doctors recommend that you hold off on HRT and consider using a low-dose oral contraceptive pill instead, as long as you do not smoke. The estrogen and progestin contained in oral contraceptives will relieve your hot flashes, regulate your menstrual cycle, and control the irregular bleeding that can occur during perimenopause. The amounts of estrogen in the low-dose pill are actually more potent than the dose commonly used for HRT after menopause and will also protect against unintended pregnancy.

If you decide to use an oral contraceptive, regular menstrual cycles will continue, even when you reach menopause. The FSH blood test discussed in Chapter 2 (see page 20) will tell you if menopause has occurred. You are advised against taking low-dose oral contraceptives if you smoke or have a history of breast cancer or blood clots. When used to relieve perimenopausal symptoms, oral contraceptives have the added benefit of providing contraception, which may be of particular benefit to sexually active women with a history of irregular cycles.

• **Vaginal symptoms.** Before menopause, one of the actions of estrogen is to keep the vaginal lining thick, elastic, and well lubricated. When estrogen levels drop, the vaginal lining becomes thinner, drier, and less elastic. The vagina is then more likely to become sore or irritated. HRT can alleviate these symptoms.

If your goal is to relieve vaginal dryness alone, vaginal estrogen therapy may be the best thing for you. These creams tend to be more effective at treating the vagina directly than nonvaginal treatments. But even with the cream, you may find it takes a few weeks before treatment starts to work. You also need to be aware that the amount of estrogen cream used to treat vaginal dryness is not absorbed in amounts sufficient to protect women against heart disease or to help prevent osteoporosis. You are advised to take progestin along with the cream to lower your risk of endometrial cancer.

There is also an estrogen-releasing ring available that is placed in the vagina, much like a diaphragm, where it slowly releases minute amounts of estrogen that restore the vaginal lining and its ability to lubricate itself. The ring must be replaced every 3 months and does not require that you take progestin therapy.

• **Emotional symptoms.** While menopause itself does not cause emotional problems, its symptoms may. Hot flashes, night sweats, decreased libido, and other symptoms can all take their toll on your emotional well-being. Fatigue, nervousness, and irritability are not uncommon in menopausal women. HRT can help restore your sense of well-being by treating the symptoms of menopause. However, emotional distress that goes beyond the normal sadness that accompanies major life events is probably better treated in other ways. See Chapter 7 for more information about managing stress.

THE DRAWBACKS OF HORMONE REPLACEMENT THERAPY

As with all medications, HRT may have side effects. Estrogen may cause nausea, bloating, breast tenderness, and headaches. More women experience side effects from progestin. The higher the progestin dose, the greater the chance of water retention, bloating, irritability, mood swings, and anxiety. The withdrawal bleeding that often follows each cycle of progestin is the most frequent reason women stop.

Although the side effects of HRT vary from woman to woman, the following are the most commonly reported:

- **Withdrawal periods.** Bleeding is a major reason women object to HRT. Most women look forward to the end of menstruation. Irregular bleeding may also cause some women to worry that they have cancer. For this reason, there are now different regimens (continuous combined therapy, for example) that allow you to avoid withdrawal bleeding.

- **Premenstrual syndrome–like symptoms.** Some possible unpleasant side effects of HRT include such premenstrual syndrome (PMS)–like symptoms as depression, irritability, bloating, and breast tenderness caused by the progestin. Estrogen can also cause fluid retention and bloating, as well as swollen, sore breasts.

You may be able to find relief from these symptoms by trying a different form or regimen. Or you may want to talk to your doctor about decreasing your progestin dosage to the bare minimum required to get the benefits you seek. The importance of working with your doctor to find relief from these uncomfortable symptoms cannot be overemphasized.

- **Skin irritation.** Transdermal skin patches can sometimes cause itching and temporary redness under the patch. Vaginal creams are also occasionally allergenic. If irritation is a problem, talk to your doctor about trying another method. In addition to irritation, some hormones can cause acnelike skin problems.

Often, this problem subsides when the hormone dosage is reduced or the hormone is discontinued.

• **Headaches.** Estrogen may trigger migraines in women who have a history of migraines related to their menstrual cycle. For these women, doctors often recommend taking estrogen and progestin continuously.

• **Facial hair and voice deepening.** Testosterone has caused the appearance of facial hair and oily skin in some women. These symptoms will disappear when the testosterone is stopped.

THE RISKS OF HORMONE REPLACEMENT THERAPY

Some women who have conditions such as breast cancer may not be able to take HRT and must use other measures for relief of symptoms and prevention of health problems such as heart disease and osteoporosis. Many women who can use hormones choose not to because they are worried about the possibility of breast cancer. Additional research will clarify the long-term risks of HRT and make it easier for women to make informed decisions.

Hormone Replacement Therapy and Breast Cancer

Breast cancer, along with lung cancer, is a major cause of death today for women between the ages of 40 and 65, and the rate at which it occurs is increasing. One in nine women will get some form of breast cancer. The issue of HRT and breast cancer is confusing because of conflicting research findings. Some studies have shown that the long-term use of HRT may be one factor related to the occurrence of breast cancer, but other studies show that there is no correlation. The relationship between HRT and breast cancer is still under investigation.

One study that found a possible connection between estrogen and breast cancer is the Nurses Health Study. The study, which has followed 122,000 nurses since 1976, has shown that the risk of breast cancer goes up slightly with the long-term use of estrogen. More specifically, the study demonstrated that after 5 to 10 years of estrogen therapy, there is a 2 percent to 3 percent increase in breast cancer risk over the average. In other words, if 12 of 100 women are at risk of getting breast cancer without using estrogen, 14 to 15 women are at risk of getting the disease after using estrogen for more than 10 years.

The relationship between progestin and breast cancer is even less clear. As with estrogen, most studies have shown that progestin has no effect on the risk for breast cancer; other studies suggest that progestin may increase breast cancer risk; still other studies demonstrate that progestin may actually reduce the risk of breast cancer. At this time, scientists do not think that progestin, taken for 5 years or less, increases breast cancer risk.

There are some important issues to consider in regard to HRT and breast cancer. First, it is thought that women who take estrogen for less than 10 years may have no increased risk of breast cancer. The risk seems to go up slightly with longer use. Second, it is thought that high doses of estrogen used in the past may be to blame. Many doctors now begin HRT with the lowest dosages possible and work from there. Also, the type of estrogen used may affect a woman's risk.

Researchers have pointed out that despite the increased risk

BREAST SELF-EXAMINATION

It is vital for every woman to examine her breasts regularly and to see her doctor as soon as possible if she finds a breast lump.

All women should perform a breast self-examination once a month and be examined by a doctor yearly. It is helpful to examine your breasts while you are lying down or in the bathtub or shower with soap on your fingers. Put your hand behind your head on the side you are examining. Remember that most breast lumps are not cancer, but all should be professionally evaluated. The current recommendation is for women to have a baseline mammogram at age 40 and then to have a regular mammogram every 1 or 2 years until age 50, when they should begin having mammograms every year. The frequency at which your doctor will recommend you have mammograms before 50 will depend on your risk of developing breast cancer.

There are many steps you can take to help prevent breast cancer. Eliminating caffeine may help decrease breast lumpiness (but not cancer), and a low-fat, high-fiber diet that includes plenty of vegetables may reduce the risk of breast cancer for some women.

---

of breast cancer with HRT, 10 times more women die of heart disease than breast cancer, and hormone use gives significant protection from heart attacks.

When weighing the risks of breast cancer against the benefits of HRT, each woman needs to review her health history and talk with her doctor.

Hormone Replacement Therapy and Uterine Cancer

Many women stopped using estrogen in the late 1970s because it was found that it increased the risk of endometrial cancer (cancer of the lining of the uterus). Since then, it has been found that

Breast self-examination

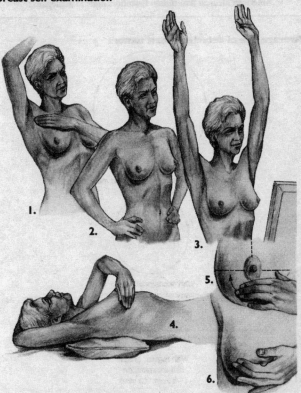

1. Stand before a mirror. Look and feel for any lumps, depressions, or differences in texture. **2.** Notice how your breasts look now (especially the nipples) so you can note future changes. **3.** Lift your arms above your head and look for swelling or dimpling in the breasts. **4.** Lie on your back with a pillow under your right shoulder and your right arm behind your head. Divide your breast into four imaginary segments, with the nipple as center. **5.** Flatten the fingers of your left hand and make firm, circular motions over each segment, feeling for lumps or tenderness. After examining the upper, outer segment, guide your hand toward your armpit and press down firmly in all directions. **6.** Carefully feel the nipple for changes in size and shape. Squeeze the nipple to check for discharge. Reverse position and examine your left breast with your right hand (steps **4** through **6**).

Average size of detected breast tumors

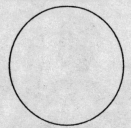

By chance (1½ inches; 38 mm)

With occasional breast
self-examination (1 inch; 25 mm)

With regular breast
self-examination
(½ inch; 13 mm)

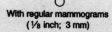

With regular mammograms
(⅛ inch; 3 mm)

The average size of cancerous breast tumors when they are detected varies significantly, according to the method of detection. The average tumor found on a regular mammogram is about 12 times smaller than the average tumor found by chance.

including progestin in the hormone regimen actually reduces this risk. In fact, the risk of endometrial cancer is lower for women taking combined estrogen–progestin therapy than it is for women who are not taking HRT. Some endometrial cancer risk remains, however, if women are not prescribed progestin for an adequate time each month or if women neglect to take it. Be sure to ask your doctor for a complete explanation of all drugs you are prescribed, including their risks, benefits, and proper dosages.

Aside from lack of progestin, other factors, such as obesity (being 20 percent or more over one's ideal body weight), increase a woman's risk of endometrial cancer. Obesity increases endometrial cancer risk because of the increased amount of natural estrogen formed in the body's fat cells. If you are obese, you should be especially careful to include at least a 12-day course of progestin monthly to prevent excess growth of the endometrium and help protect against endometrial cancer.

Hormone Replacement Therapy and Thromboembolic Disease

Thromboembolic disease refers to any condition in which the body is more likely to form blood clots. It includes a number of conditions, including stroke and heart attacks if they are caused by a clot that blocks an already narrowed artery.

Early high-dose oral contraceptives increased the risk of blood clots, especially in older women who smoked cigarettes. High doses of estrogen increase clotting factors. The higher the dose of estrogen, the higher the risk of clotting. If you smoke, the risk is even higher. However, the doses of estrogen used in postmenopausal HRT are much lower than those used in contemporary birth control pills. For this reason, if a woman does not currently have a blood clot or inflammation of deep leg veins, she may use postmenopausal HRT.

Hormone Replacement Therapy and Uterine Fibroids

Uterine fibroids are benign overgrowths of the smooth muscle of the uterus. Their growth may be stimulated by high doses of estrogen, such as those the body makes in pregnancy. Ordinarily, fibroid tumors shrink after menopause because of decreased estrogen levels, and they rarely cause additional problems. Commonly prescribed doses of HRT are so low that they typically do not cause growth of these tumors. For most women with fibroids who take HRT at or after menopause, fibroids continue to shrink.

Testosterone's Risks

Many doctors are now prescribing testosterone along with estrogen–progestin therapy for certain postmenopausal women. These women frequently experience an enhanced libido and an improved sense of well-being.

Some women taking testosterone have experienced side effects, such as acne, facial hair, weight gain, or oily skin. These side effects are quickly reversed when the testosterone therapy is reduced or stopped.

MAKING THE DECISION

Balancing the short-term and long-term health benefits of HRT against its potential risks has been a source of uncertainty for many women. It is important for every woman to understand her options and the full range of the benefits and risks of HRT.

Begin With a Checkup

A physical examination and screening tests taken around the time you reach menopause can give you a better idea of your health profile and how you can benefit from HRT. It can also help determine which hormone doses and treatment regimen might be best for you.

This pretherapy evaluation also gives you an opportunity to review your overall health. Menopause is an excellent time to address health issues that you might have let slip for too long. It is a time when you can begin to take control and potentially avoid some of the health problems so many women face in their later years.

The examinations used to evaluate whether you will benefit from HRT vary, depending on your doctor and your perceived risks for certain health problems. The following are those that most doctors choose to perform on menopausal women:

• **A complete medical history and physical examination.** A complete physical examination typically includes a blood pressure test, a breast and pelvic examination, and a guaiac test, which checks for blood in the stools.

• **Screening tests.** Screening tests include a Pap smear for the detection of cervical cancer and a rectal exam for colon cancer. All women should have a Pap smear every 6 to 12 months, depending on their doctor's recommendation. The current recommendation is for women to have a baseline mammogram at age

40 and then to have a regular mammogram every 1 or 2 years until age 50, when they should begin having mammograms every year. The frequency at which your doctor will recommend you have mammograms before age 50 will depend on your risk of developing breast cancer.

• **A lipid profile.** A lipid profile gives you a picture of the levels of different types of fat in your blood. Slightly abnormal levels can be controlled through diet and exercise, but more abnormal levels may need to be treated with medication.

• **Diabetes screen.** A test to check blood glucose (sugar) levels may be necessary if there is a family history of diabetes or if you have any symptoms of the disease, such as unexplained weight loss, excessive thirst, or frequent urination.

• **Endometrial biopsy.** If you are experiencing unexplained vaginal bleeding, an endometrial biopsy (removal of cells from the uterus for microscopic examination) should be performed to check for cancer or precancerous tissue in the uterus.

• **Bone mass densitometry.** If you have risk factors for osteoporosis, a bone densitometry test such as dual energy X-ray absorptiometry (DEXA) or dual photon absorptiometry (DPA) measures the strength and density of your bone mass. For more information on bone density testing, see page 58.

Who Should Avoid Hormone Replacement Therapy?

Some women may not be able to take HRT because of a health condition such as the following. However, it is essential to discuss your options with your doctor.

• **A history of breast cancer.** If you have breast cancer, HRT is not currently recommended by most doctors. However, a family history of breast cancer, even in a close relative such as a mother or a sister, does not rule out taking HRT.

• **A history of advanced endometrial cancer.** If you have had endometrial cancer that was diagnosed at an advanced stage, your doctor may recommend against taking HRT.

• **An active blood-clotting disorder.** Women who use estrogen-containing oral contraceptives are at a slightly increased risk of developing clots in the veins of their legs that can travel to the lungs. This risk has been shown to increase if the woman is over age 35 and smokes. However, the low doses of estrogen commonly prescribed as part of postmenopausal HRT do not carry a similar increased risk, as long as a woman does not already have an active inflammation or other disease in her deep leg veins.

• **Unexplained vaginal bleeding.** Any unusual bleeding can be an indication of abnormal tissue inside the uterus, perhaps even cancer. Report any unexplained vaginal bleeding to your doctor before starting HRT.

• **Liver disease.** If you have chronic or active liver disease, such as hepatitis, cirrhosis, or bile problems, your doctor may recommend that you postpone HRT until after a full evaluation of your liver. Liver enzyme blood tests can evaluate your liver function, and since hormone pills are metabolized in the liver, the dosage may need to be adjusted accordingly. A nonoral form of estrogen, such as the skin patch, may be a better choice for you.

LIFE WITH HORMONE REPLACEMENT THERAPY

If you decide to try HRT, regular visits to your doctor should be part of your health-care routine. Follow-up visits, every 6 to 12 months (depending on your doctor's recommendation), are helpful to fine-tune your regimen and monitor changes in your hormone levels.

While you are taking HRT, it may be a good idea to keep a diary of any symptoms you notice in order to better inform your doctor. Call your doctor as soon as possible if any of the following occur:

- You have unexpected vaginal bleeding
- You find a breast lump or have unrelieved breast tenderness
- You have an unexpected vaginal discharge
- You experience severe headaches, chest pain, shortness of breath, or swelling or pain in one or both legs

6

Other Medications

In addition to prescribing a healthy lifestyle and hormone replacement therapy (HRT), many doctors prescribe other medications to help treat the symptoms of menopause or the health risks associated with it. Some of these drugs lower cholesterol levels, others work to prevent or halt osteoporosis, and still others work to relieve hot flashes.

Any medication may produce side effects. Be sure you know what the drug's possible side effects are and what to do if you experience them.

Below is a summary of the drugs most often prescribed today to women who are dealing with menopause.

CALCIUM METABOLISM

To understand how some of the drugs described here work in fighting osteoporosis, take a closer look at how calcium is metabolized in the body. *Metabolism* is a word used to describe the chemical activities that take place in your body, such as burning food for energy and creating chemicals your body needs from other substances. This process is controlled by hormones, special chemicals produced by your endocrine system (and other organs) that work together to regulate your metabolism continuously and rapidly.

Your body works to keep the level of calcium in your blood constant by balancing the amount of calcium that is absorbed with the amount that is lost. This process is called calcium metabolism. Three hormones are needed to balance the level of calcium in your blood. Parathyroid hormone, secreted by the parathyroid glands, causes your body to release calcium from your bones when the level of calcium in your blood is too low. Another hormone, calcitonin, secreted by the thyroid gland, works against parathyroid hormone when the level of calcium in your blood is too high. A third hormone, calcitriol (a form of vitamin D), is stored in the liver and kidneys when inactive and works with parathyroid hormones when it is needed. A finely tuned interaction between parathyroid hormone, calcitonin, and calcitriol is vital to maintaining a stable level of calcium in your blood.

BISPHOSPHONATES

Two bisphosphonates are currently on the market for the treatment and prevention of osteoporosis: etidronate (brand name, Didronel) and alendronate (brand name, Fosamax). More drugs in this family are expected to be on the market soon.

Drug Action

Bisphosphonates are drugs that inhibit bone breakdown and slow bone removal. They act by binding to osteoclasts (the cells that take calcium out of bone) and preventing them from functioning. They effectively decrease bone loss in postmenopausal women and even help women build up their bones.

Alendronate is approved not only for the treatment of osteoporosis but also for its prevention in women who are at increased risk.

Side Effects

Alendronate's major side effect is the possibility of reflux (regurgitation of acid fluid from the stomach) of the esophagus when it is not taken in exactly the right way. Alendronate must be taken on an empty stomach for maximum absorption. The manufacturer strongly recommends taking it with a full glass of water (8 ounces) first thing in the morning and then waiting at least 30 minutes, and preferably 1 hour, before eating any food, drinking any beverage, or taking any other medication. To minimize the risk of reflux irritation to the esophagus, the manufacturer instructs women not to lie down for at least 30 minutes after taking the medication.

Other side effects of bisphosphonates include nausea, gastrointestinal cramping, difficulty swallowing, bloating, constipation, diarrhea, gas, and an altered sense of taste.

There are currently no long-term studies on the potential additive benefits of using alendronate with estrogen. Estrogen is still considered the first-choice therapy for osteoporosis, owing to its added benefits in reducing cardiovascular disease, Alzheimer's disease, and colon cancer.

CALCITONIN

Calcitonin is a hormone made by the thyroid gland that inhibits bone breakdown. Today, there is a synthetic form of calcitonin (brand names, Calcimar, Cibacalcin, and Miacalcin).

Drug Action

Calcitonin helps to block bone loss. It is used for the treatment of postmenopausal osteoporosis in women who are more than 5 years past menopause and who have low bone mass compared with women before menopause. It is also recommended for women who cannot take estrogen.

In women who are at least 5 years beyond menopause, calcitonin appears to slow bone loss, increase spinal bone density, and, according to some reports, relieve the pain associated with bone fractures. The drug may also reduce the risk of spinal and hip fractures. Calcitonin also helps to control the level of calcium in the blood. In addition to treatment for osteoporosis, it is used to treat Paget's disease (abnormal bone growth leading to deformities) and hypercalcemia (abnormally high calcium blood levels).

Right now, researchers do not know whether calcitonin builds bone or just prevents its loss. It is also not clear whether the effects of calcitonin persist beyond 2 or 3 years. In 2-year studies, it has been found to increase bone density by 5 percent when taken with calcium.

Calcitonin is not absorbed very well when taken orally. Therefore, it is administered as a nasal spray to be used twice a day. It appears to be especially helpful for women over age 65. The only reported side effect thus far is nasal or sinus irritation.

Calcitonin can also be taken by injection, given by either you or your doctor. If you are injecting it yourself, it is important that you follow all instructions carefully so that you inject it correctly. The drug should be injected under the skin or into a muscle, not into a vein. You can minimize the potential side effects of nausea, vomiting, and skin flushing by taking the injection at bedtime. You must be careful not to use the injection solution if it has changed color or has particles floating in it.

If you are taking calcitonin for postmenopausal bone loss, you should be sure your diet provides enough calcium (at least 1,500 milligrams per day) and vitamin D (400 international units per day) to help in its effects on your bones.

Side Effects

More common side effects of calcitonin use may include inflamed skin at the injection site (if injected), nausea, and vomiting. Less common side effects may include flushed face, flushed hands, allergic reaction, and rashes.

If you experience any side effects or if they change in intensity, inform your doctor as soon as possible.

CALCITRIOL

As we have noted, vitamin D is an important addition to calcium because it improves the body's ability to absorb and use calcium effectively. Calcitriol (brand names, Calcijex and Rocaltrol) is a hormonally active form of vitamin D.

Drug Action

Taken orally, calcitriol slows bone resorption and promotes a dramatic increase in the absorption of calcium by the intestine and prompt repair of diseased bone. Most doctors agree that the improvement in bone strength and density results from the alleviation of any calcium deficiency. Calcium is resorbed from the digestive tract, but bone formation is not enhanced with calcitriol.

Side Effects

Some studies have shown that high doses of calcitriol are associated with side effects such as hypercalcemia (an excess of calcium in the blood) and a deterioration in kidney function. More long-term studies are needed to determine the safety and effectiveness of this drug.

RALOXIFENE

Raloxifene (brand name, Evista) is a medication that helps prevent osteoporosis. It is a type of drug known as a selective estrogen receptor modulator (SERM), a so-called designer estrogen. Raloxifene is prescribed only for women who are past menopause and who are not taking hormone replacement therapy. Other drugs of this type are currently being developed.

Drug Action

Raloxifene acts like estrogen on bone tissue, although it may not be as effective as estrogen. In most women, raloxifene stops the bone loss that often occurs after menopause, helping to maintain bone strength. However, the drug rebuilds bone tissue to a lesser extent than estrogen does, and it is not yet known whether the drug prevents fractures. Although its benefits to the cardiovascular system are not completely understood, research has shown that raloxifene lowers blood levels of LDL ("bad") cholesterol but has no effect on blood levels of HDL ("good") cholesterol.

Unlike estrogen, raloxifene does not relieve symptoms of menopause such as hot flashes, night sweats, mood swings, or insomnia. Raloxifene has no effect on breast, vaginal, or uterine tissues. Preliminary evidence also suggests that raloxifene may help prevent breast cancer. **Warning:** If you experience breast pain or swelling or vaginal bleeding while taking this medication, see your doctor as soon as possible.

Side Effects

A major side effect of raloxifene is an increase in the occurrence of hot flashes, usually during the first six months of taking the drug. These hot flashes are generally mild. Another possible side effect is leg cramps.

Special Precautions

Do not take raloxifene if you are taking hormone replacement therapy. Do not take raloxifene if you are pregnant or if you could become pregnant, because the drug can harm a fetus. Also, raloxifene is not recommended for women who have had liver disease.

Women taking raloxifene have a slightly increased risk of deep vein thrombosis (formation of blood clots in deep-lying veins, usually in the legs). You should not take this drug if you have or have had blood clots or if you will be immobile for a long period of time (such as after having surgery). **Warning:** Blood clots are a serious health problem that can lead to disability or even death. If you experience symptoms such as pain in the calves or leg swelling, sudden chest pain, shortness of breath, coughing up blood, or blurred vision, call 911 or your local emergency number, or go directly to the nearest hospital emergency department.

Because this drug is effective only if you take it as prescribed, be sure to follow your doctor's instructions carefully.

SODIUM FLUORIDE

Sodium fluoride is a naturally occurring mineral found in trace amounts in seafood, vegetables, meats, cereal, fruits, and tea. It is often added to drinking water.

Drug Action

It has long been known that fluoride helps prevent dental cavities. A 1960 study also found a higher incidence of osteoporosis among people with low levels of fluoride in their drinking water. Several other studies showed that fluoride actually stimulates the formation of new bone, although the precise mechanism is unknown.

One problem is that bone tissue formed while taking sodium fluoride is not as strong as normal bones. There have been several reports of increased fractures of the hip.

Newer, slow-release forms of sodium fluoride are associated with lower blood levels of fluoride and may be associated with fewer fractures. (Some common brand names include Fluoritab, Fluorodex, and Luride.) Fluoride might work better in combination with other therapies, particularly estrogen therapy. This way, the new bone being formed by fluoride will be enough (boosted by estrogen therapy) for calcium to adhere to.

Side Effects

Another problem with fluoride therapy is side effects. The most common are gastrointestinal problems, such as stomach pains, nausea, vomiting, and diarrhea. These side effects are minimized by using time-release preparations or coated sodium-fluoride tablets.

Sodium-fluoride tablets are widely available without a prescription at local pharmacies. However, until more is known about the effectiveness of fluoride in the treatment of osteoporosis, take fluoride tablets only on your doctor's recommendation (especially if you have high blood pressure).

TAMOXIFEN

Tamoxifen (brand name, Nolvadex) is commonly used to treat women with breast cancer. It is typically prescribed for 5 years and then discontinued. Tamoxifen is used to delay the recurrence of breast cancer following appropriate treatment and to combat metastatic (cancer that spreads to another part of the body) breast cancer as an alternative to radiation or removal of the ovaries.

Drug Action

Tamoxifen tablets block the action of estrogen by binding to estrogen receptor sites on cells. Tamoxifen thus competes with estrogen for receptor sites in breast tissue where the estrogen normally exerts its actions. The result is a decrease in the growth of breast tissue and possibly of breast cancer tissue. Researchers were once concerned that this antiestrogenic (estrogen blocking) effect might be harmful to bones. They found, to their surprise, that tamoxifen acts differently in bone tissues. Instead of blocking estrogen in bones, the drug acts like estrogen on bone, slowing bone loss and preserving bone mass. Research has found that in women receiving tamoxifen, bone of the lumbar spine is preserved and even increases. More research is needed before tamoxifen can be used to treat osteoporosis, but so far the results are encouraging.

Typically, most women respond well to tamoxifen if tests show that their breast tumors are sensitive to the effects of estrogen. If they develop resistance to tamoxifen, the tumor will begin to recur. However, for many women who no longer respond to tamoxifen, other effective hormonal agents can be used. These alternative drugs usually work for a while, after which the woman again may develop resistance. Tamoxifen tends to be given as "first-line" therapy because it has significantly fewer side effects than other drugs.

Tamoxifen should be taken exactly as prescribed. Do not stop taking the medication without first consulting your doctor.

Side Effects

Side effects of tamoxifen are usually mild and rarely require that you stop taking the drug. The most common side effects are hot flashes and nausea and/or vomiting. The side effects are related to tamoxifen's antiestrogenic activity, although the drug is known to have some estrogenic (estrogen promoting) effects as well. Overall, the incidence of hormone-related side effects is much lower in postmenopausal women. In premenopausal women, tamoxifen may produce symptoms similar to menopause. Menstrual irregularities, vaginal bleeding, and vaginal dryness or itching have all been reported. Other gastrointestinal problems including loss of appetite, constipation, and diarrhea; edema (water retention) and weight gain have also been reported. If any of these side effects develop or change in intensity, inform your doctor as soon as possible. Only your doctor can determine if it is safe for you to continue taking tamoxifen.

Special Precautions

Tamoxifen use may be linked to an increased risk of thromboembolic disease (which causes blood-clotting problems) and changes in the endometrial layer of the uterus (including polyps, hyperplasia, and, rarely, cancer). It is for this reason that if you are taking tamoxifen, you need to be aware of the early warning signs of these problems.

Warning: If you experience abnormal vaginal bleeding; leg swelling, pain, and warmth; or abrupt shortness of breath, chest pain, and cough, with spitting up of blood, it is vital to contact your doctor immediately. Periodic pelvic examinations are very important for catching early any problems involving the endometrium.

On rare occasions, tamoxifen may produce hypercalcemia (an abnormally high level of calcium in the blood). Symptoms of hypercalcemia include muscle pain and weakness and loss of appetite. If you experience any of these symptoms, notify your doctor as soon as possible.

Breast Cancer Prevention Trial

A study by the National Cancer Institute (NCI) has shown that tamoxifen can prevent breast cancer in high-risk women who do not already have the disease. The study, called the Breast Cancer Prevention Trial, began in 1992 and ended in 1998, more than one year ahead of schedule because the drug was found to be more effective than anticipated. In all, 13,388 women age 35 and older took part in the study.

The study found a 45-percent lower incidence of breast cancer among the women who took tamoxifen compared with the group of women who took a placebo (an inactive pill). Also, the women who took tamoxifen had fewer fractures of the hip, spine, and wrist.

However, the study also showed an increased risk of serious side effects from the drug, especially in women over age 50. Side effects include endometrial cancer (cancer of the lining of the uterus), pulmonary embolism (blood clots in the lungs), and deep-vein thrombosis (blood clots in major veins, usually in the legs).

For many at-risk women, the benefits of taking tamoxifen outweigh the risks. Women who are at increased risk of breast cancer can now work with their physicians to decide whether they should take tamoxifen, based on their individual risks and personal preferences.

CLONIDINE

Clonidine (brand name, Catapres), usually prescribed to treat high blood pressure, may also lessen hot flashes, but not as effectively as estrogen. So clonidine is not commonly prescribed to treat hot flashes.

Drug Action

A neurotransmitter is a chemical that sends nerve impulses in the body. Clonidine blocks the neurotransmitter norepinephrine (which is elevated when hot flashes occur), and it appears to stabilize the temperature-regulating center of the hypothalamus. Clonidine may also block the dilation (widening) of blood vessels in the arms and legs, which occurs during a hot flash.

In the largest studies, clonidine reduced the number and frequency of hot flashes among women who took it, depending on the dosage. Higher doses were more effective, but higher doses were also related to bothersome side effects, including dry mouth and dizziness.

Clonidine works best when delivered via a skin patch worn on the shoulder. The skin patch is changed once a week. Clonidine is also available in oral and injectable forms.

Side Effects

The side effects of clonidine include dry mouth, nausea, fatigue, headaches, and dizziness.

ERGOTAMINE, BELLADONNA ALKALOIDS, AND PHENOBARBITAL

Ergotamine, belladonna alkaloids, and phenobarbital combination (brand name, Bellergal-S) is a mild sedative preparation that is occasionally prescribed to treat symptoms of menopause.

Drug Action

This combination of medications relieves some symptoms of menopause—hot flashes, sweating, restlessness, and insomnia—in about half of the women who take it, and is a good choice for women with breast cancer, who are usually advised not to take estrogen. However, it is not an effective treatment for menopause-related health problems such as osteoporosis.

Ergotamine, belladonna alkaloids, and phenobarbital combination is available in a timed-release tablet that can be taken once before bedtime, or if symptoms are severe, once in the morning and again at night. Because phenobarbital can be addicting, the drug is used only for short periods of time.

Side Effects

Side effects of this medication include dizziness and drowsiness. Other common side effects include dry mouth and constipation.

COMPLEMENTARY THERAPIES

Alternative or complementary practitioners may recommend that you take anise, the herb black cohosh, and licorice to promote estrogen production in your body. (**Warning**: Licorice is a stimulant; do not take it if you have high blood pressure.) They may also recommend that you take evening primrose oil supplements to help reduce the severity of menopausal symptoms. However, it is important to note that mainstream medicine does not endorse these therapies and that there is no scientific proof regarding their safety and effectiveness. Talk to your doctor if you decide to take them.

7

A Healthy Lifestyle

GETTING FIT, STAYING FIT

Many of the health problems we blame on aging are actually the result of physical inactivity. But the good news is that if you exercise regularly, you can prevent, slow, or even reverse many of these changes. Among the many benefits of regular exercise are a reduced risk of heart disease, osteoporosis, and colon cancer; successful weight control; improved appearance; improved balance and coordination; decreased pain from many health problems; improved emotional well-being; and better, more restful sleep.

THE MANY BENEFITS OF EXERCISE

When you exercise regularly, you and your body reap many rewards, including the following:

- Your cells receive more oxygen, which improves blood circulation, creates energy, and improves your ability to handle stress.
- Exercise can help you deal with depression and improve your sense of well-being.
- Improved health will add years to your life.
- Constipation may decrease or disappear.
- You sleep better.
- You have an easier time controlling your weight, because regular exercise helps to burn calories, diminish your appetite, and speed your body's metabolism.
- Your bones become stronger, helping prevent osteoporosis.
- Your risk of heart disease declines.
- Lung function and endurance improve.
- Your chances of getting colon cancer decrease.
- Your risk of developing adult-onset diabetes decreases, as exercise improves your body's ability to use sugar in the blood.
- Joint stiffness, arthritis, and low-back pain lessen.

Heart Disease Prevention

Heart disease is the leading cause of death among women over age 65. The type of heart disease most often seen in older women involves coronary arteries that are narrowed or blocked by deposits of cholesterol. A diet high in fat and cholesterol, cigarette smoking, and lack of exercise are the likely causes of heart disease. Having a healthy lifestyle is the best way to reduce your risk of heart disease. And regular exercise is an important part of a healthy lifestyle.

Regular aerobic exercise (see page 123) does great things for your heart: it makes your heart a more efficient pump, causing more blood to circulate with each beat, thus sending more oxygen to your muscles. As a result, your heart, lungs, and muscles work more efficiently while you exercise.

When you first start a walking program, for example, you may feel tired after walking only a short distance. But after a month of regular, brisk walking your heart and lungs become conditioned, so you can easily take longer and longer walks. Just as your arm and leg muscles get stronger the more you use them, so does your heart muscle. Regular aerobic exercise makes your heart a stronger, more efficient pump.

One way to determine the condition of your heart is to check your resting heart rate by taking your pulse first thing in the morning before you get out of bed. Check your pulse at your wrist or at the side of your neck using your index and middle fingers. Count the beats for 1 minute. If your heart is conditioned, it will beat slowly while at rest, because it will be stronger and send more oxygen-rich blood throughout the body with each beat. As you become more fit, your resting pulse rate drops.

While it may be easy to see how regular exercise improves the condition of the heart, it may be difficult to understand how it prevents deposits of fat and cholesterol from clogging the blood vessels. Exercise accomplishes this in a couple of ways. First, exercise encourages the formation of new, tiny capillaries to supply the heart. Second, it makes the blood flow less sluggish and less likely to clot. It is for these reasons that if you exercise, you are less likely to have heart disease or stroke. In addition, regular exercise raises the level of "good" high density lipoprotein (HDL) cholesterol and lowers the level of "bad" low density lipoprotein (LDL) cholesterol in the blood. Studies have also shown that regular exercise helps lower high blood pressure.

In addition to its heart benefits, exercise helps you to develop endurance so that you have more energy throughout the day. When you climb a flight of stairs, run to catch a bus, or play tennis with a friend, you will feel better.

Before you begin an exercise program, talk to your doctor. This is especially important if you have a history of heart disease, diabetes, high blood pressure, or chest pain. A checkup is very important if you are middle-aged, have been inactive, and plan to start an exercise program.

Note that any exercise is better for your heart than no exercise at all. Your heart will benefit even if your exercise is spread out in short segments (10 to 20 minutes) throughout the day. Swimming, bicycling, brisk walking, gardening, housecleaning, and dancing are all good choices. Try to fit some brisk walking into your day, every day—walk to the store, walk to the mailbox, and use the stairs instead of the elevator. If you are physically challenged, you can often find an activity, such as swimming or water exercise, that will get your heart pumping.

Effects of Exercise on Bone

In general, when it comes to exercise, what is good for your heart is good for your bones. Regular exercise can go a long way toward preventing osteoporosis. A number of studies have shown that women can reduce the effects of osteoporosis by exercising on a regular basis. And it is important to stress the *regular* in *regular exercise.* As soon as you stop exercising for as little as a week, bone density will gradually begin to decline. Bone density will increase when you start exercising again.

Because there is no cure for osteoporosis, the best way to fight it is with prevention, and exercise is vital to preventing osteoporosis. Women who are inactive quickly lose calcium from their bones. Conversely, active women who regularly perform weight-bearing exercises develop thicker, stronger bones.

Weight-bearing exercises are those that put stress on the large muscles of the lower body. Brisk walking, dancing, or jogging are some good examples. Studies have shown that postmenopausal women who consistently walk a mile or more every day lose bone more slowly than sedentary women.

Along with bone tissue, women tend to lose muscle strength as they age. Regular exercise can help keep a woman's muscles strong. After all, whatever builds muscle will build bones. Muscle-strengthening exercises for the back, abdomen, shoulders, and arms are important to helping prevent spinal osteoporosis. In fact, strength training for people over age 70 is considered the best way to prolong independence. Gardening or lifting weights are good choices.

Even if you are confined to bed, you need to exercise, because bones rapidly weaken if you become inactive. If you spend the day at home ill, remember to move around as well as rest. Get up every few hours, stretch, walk, and work your muscles gently. Your recovery will be easier, and your bones will remain strong.

Weight Control

If you have ever tried to lose weight or to maintain your weight, you know how difficult it can be if you do not exercise regularly.

FIND YOUR HEALTHY WEIGHT

Compare your actual weight to the recommended healthy weight range for your height and frame size (most women have a medium frame).

Note: Heights shown are in feet and inches, without shoes; weights shown are in pounds, without clothes.

| | WEIGHT | | |
HEIGHT	SMALL FRAME	MEDIUM FRAME	LARGE FRAME
5′	98–106	103–115	111–127
5′1″	101–109	106–118	114–130
5′2″	104–112	109–122	117–134
5′3″	107–115	112–126	121–138
5′4″	110–119	116–131	125–142
5′5″	114–123	120–135	129–146
5′6″	118–127	124–139	133–150
5′7″	122–131	128–143	137–154
5′8″	126–136	132–147	141–159
5′9″	130–140	136–151	145–164
5′10″	134–144	140–155	149–169

If you have any questions about your ideal weight, talk to your doctor.

Your body senses when you are dieting and lowers its resting metabolic rate. In other words, when you start to eat less, your body makes up for it by slowing down and conserving energy by burning calories more slowly. (This is to help keep you from starving to death if you are lost in the wilderness.)

However, if you increase your body's need for calories through exercise, your resting metabolic rate will remain stable or may even increase. Therefore, a weight-reduction program that combines both exercise and diet is more effective and is more likely to result in successful maintenance of weight loss.

But be aware that successful weight loss through diet and exercise is a slow process. In reality, there are no quick fixes. The best types of exercises for weight loss are those that use up large amounts of calories by keeping a large percentage of the body's muscles working over an extended period of time. Bicycling, jogging, swimming, and aerobic dancing are some good examples.

Better Balance and Coordination

The more a muscle repeats an activity, the more efficient it becomes. Your body as a whole works in the same way. As you perform the same activity over time, you become better able to perform that activity. It becomes almost reflex in nature. Therefore, even if you feel awkward when you first begin an exercise program, your performance will improve over time.

Another benefit to exercise is that it may improve your coordination and balance, making it less likely that you will have a disabling fall.

Improved Emotional Well-being

Exercise has extremely beneficial effects on mood. Physical activity stimulates the brain, causing the release of substances called endorphins that help you feel good. As a result, depression and physical pain are lessened. This is the "high" that athletes experience while training intensely. Some doctors even prescribe exercise to help treat depression.

Women who have trouble sleeping often find themselves feeling irritable and fatigued during the day, and this has a negative effect on their emotional and physical health. However, women who exercise on a regular basis tend to sleep more soundly at night. If you have trouble with insomnia, prescribe yourself a bit of daily exercise. Chances are good that you will sleep better and more soundly. A good night's sleep can do wonders for your emotional health. But avoid exercising right before bedtime, which could make it difficult for you to fall asleep.

STARTING AN EXERCISE PROGRAM

Women approaching menopause have specific fitness needs that can best be met by three types of exercise: aerobic exercise, muscle strengthening, and stretching. Any of these three can be weight-bearing exercise, too, and the more weight-bearing exercises you choose, the more your bones will benefit. When you plan your exercise program, be sure to include all three types. Also, choose exercises you really enjoy and try to include them in your daily routine.

Aerobic Exercise

Aerobic means "depending on oxygen." All aerobic exercises have one thing in common: as your muscles work, they demand more oxygen. The main objective of an aerobic exercise program is to increase the amount of oxygen your body can process within a certain time.

For your workout to be aerobic, you must engage in activity

Exercises to help build your strength

If you have not been exercising regularly, or if you want to build muscle strength without using a weight machine, the following exercises are a good place to start.

The modified push-up is the best overall upper body strengthener for women. Lie face down on the floor with your palms next to your shoulders and push up with your hands, raising your upper body from your knees, keeping your back straight. Push up until your arms are almost straight (but not locked) at the elbows. Lower your body until it almost touches the floor and repeat as many times as you can without straining.

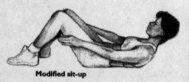

If this is too difficult for you, start with standing push-ups. Face a wall with your toes about 12 inches from the wall, arms bent, and your palms flat against the wall at shoulder height. Push away from the wall, keeping your back straight, not arched. You can increase the resistance by standing 18 inches from the wall.

Modified push-up

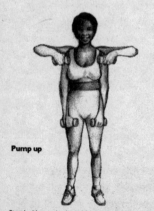

Modified sit-up

Lie on your back with your knees bent and your arms straight at your sides. Press the small of your back to the floor (to avoid straining your back). Lift your head and upper body until most of your upper back is off the floor. Hold for a count of two. Lower your body to the floor. When you can repeat the exercise 12 times without straining, increase the resistance by lifting farther off the floor, holding a light weight to your chest, or by exercising on an incline with your buttocks higher than your head.

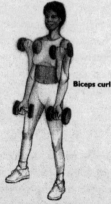

Biceps curl

Pump up

Stand with your back straight, knees slightly bent, and feet slightly apart. Hold the weights (begin with 1-pound weights) in front of your thighs, palms turned inward. Raise the weights slowly to chest level without turning your palms. Your elbows should go straight out to the sides. Lower the weights slowly to thigh level. When you can repeat the exercise 12 times without straining, increase the weights by 1 pound.

Stand with your back straight, knees slightly bent, and feet slightly apart. Hold the weights (begin with 1-pound weights) in your hands in front of your thighs, palms turned outward. Slowly bring the weights up and in toward your chest. Lower them slowly to thigh level again. When you can repeat the exercise 12 times without straining, increase the weights by 1 pound.

that works the muscles and the heart, exercise at a specified intensity, and exercise regularly. Most fitness experts say you need to work out at least three times a week to maintain your fitness level or five times a week to improve it.

How hard you exercise is up to you. One way to determine if you are working as hard as you would like to is to monitor your heart rate. As you exercise, your body's oxygen demand goes up and your heart beats faster. You want to be sure that your heart rate stays within a specified range—your training range.

First, you need to determine the training range that is right for you. Do this by taking your pulse in the middle of an aerobic workout. If the exercise has truly been aerobic, your heart rate will fall somewhere between 60 and 80 percent of your maximum heart rate (MHR), which is calculated by subtracting your age from 220. Here is an example, using a 50-year-old woman:

220 − 50 = 170 (This is the average maximum heart rate for a healthy person this age.)

170 × .60 = 102 beats per minute (If this person wants to work out at 60 percent of her maximum heart rate, this is the number of beats per minute she is to try to attain in her aerobic workout.)

170 × .80 = 136 beats per minute (This is how fast her heart should beat if she wants to work out at 80 percent of maximum.)

In this example, the woman's training range is 102 to 136 beats per minute. She wants to stay within this range as she works out aerobically. To determine your training range, simply plug in your age for the woman's age in the example.

In order to monitor your pulse while you exercise, you need a watch or clock with a second hand, and you should know what your training range is before you start. After exercising for 5 minutes, slow down just enough to read the second hand. Take your pulse, but do not stop exercising. Place your fingertips about an inch below your ear at the pulse on the side of your neck and count for 10 seconds. Multiply the number of beats you counted by 6 to get a per-minute rate. If your pulse is over your training range, slow down; if it is under, work a little harder; if it is right on, continue exercising for 20 to 30 minutes. Eventually, you will be able to tell when you are within your range, and you will not have to watch the clock.

If you are currently exercising on a regular basis, continue to exercise for the rest of your life. If you are just beginning to exercise, it is a good idea to begin with an easy activity, such as brisk walking. Take short walks at first, then gradually work your way up to at least 30 minutes per day of brisk, uninterrupted walking. You can do this all at once or divide it into two 15-minute sessions or three 10-minute sessions. Walking is an excellent form of aerobic exercise that you can maintain for the rest of your life. You can walk just about anywhere. If it is too cold or wet outside, you can exercise indoors at a recreation center or indoor shopping mall. All you really need is a good pair of walking shoes with strong arch support. If you do not like walking or want to vary your activities, other forms of exercise that are good to begin with include swimming or riding a stationary bicycle.

Muscle Strengthening

At midlife, adding weight training to your exercise program offers many benefits. While this type of exercise is not aerobic and does not reduce body fat, it can help you reverse the muscle and bone loss that comes with aging. Studies have found that fat mass increases with age, while both muscle mass and skeletal (bone) mass decline. The reduction in muscle mass may aggravate the bone loss.

Strong muscles protect the joints and help prevent exercise-related injuries. They improve the way your clothes fit and the way you feel about yourself.

When you are beginning a weight-training program, it is important to start slowly and get some expert advice. You can begin a program at home fairly inexpensively. All you need are sets of 3-pound and 5-pound dumbbells. To make progress, lift two or three times a week and wait 1 to 2 days between workouts. Brisk walking is a good activity for the days off, so that you alternate between aerobic activity and muscle strengthening.

Stretching Exercises

Stretching exercises increase flexibility and may help prevent injury. And flexibility helps make getting around a lot easier. Muscles and connective tissue lose their ability to stretch when they are not used and with aging. Joints need to move through their full range of motion regularly to maintain their flexibility. For many people, stretching reduces joint pain and low-back discomfort, improves posture, and minimizes postexercise muscle or joint soreness.

It is best to stretch muscles when they are already warm. Before you start stretching, warm up your muscles by exercising slowly. For example, warm up for jogging by walking; warm up for swimming by swinging your arms. As you warm up, the temperature of your muscles rises (hence the term *warm up*), enabling them to work more easily. Stretching before a workout may reduce your chances of injury, and stretching afterward helps to

EXERCISING YOUR OPTIONS

AEROBIC ACTIVITIES

Walking/race walking
Hiking
Jogging
Bicycling
Stationary bicycling
Rowing
Jumping rope
Swimming
Racket sports
Mowing the lawn (hand mower)
Cross-country skiing
Stair climbing
Aerobic dancing (in a class or to a video)
Step aerobics (in a class or to a video)

STRETCHING ACTIVITIES

Dancing
Yoga
Floor exercises

PLACES TO WORK OUT

Outside
At home
At a gym or health club
At a mall

fight muscle soreness and enhances muscle relaxation. So, before each workout, warm up and then stretch. After each workout, cool down and stretch again.

There is a right way and a wrong way to stretch. Stretching should be done slowly and deliberately to be effective. Rapid or jerky movements are not beneficial and may even be harmful if too much tension is placed on the muscle being stretched.

Choosing an Activity

Finding an exercise that you really enjoy takes some thought. Consider whether you want to take a class and be with people at a set time or exercise yourself on your own schedule. Do you want to exercise indoors or outside? With music or without? Do you enjoy team sports and competition? Was there any exercise you did as a child or adolescent that would be fun to take up again, like swimming, jumping rope, biking, or dancing? Consider also whether you prefer to do different exercises on different days. Perhaps you want to join a gym and work out on your lunch

GETTING A COMPLETE WORKOUT

In order to include all three types of exercise, you may have to work out for about 1 hour at least three times a week. On other days, you can skip the weight training and concentrate on stretching and aerobic exercise. Keep in mind that these are merely suggestions. Do what you enjoy and you are more likely to keep exercising. And always remember to drink plenty of water before, during, and after your workout, so that you do not become dehydrated.

Here is how a 1-hour workout session might look:

1. **Warm up (5 minutes).** Warm up before exercising by slowly stretching all of your muscles (arms, legs, chest, shoulders, abdomen). Stretching will improve flexibility, help increase blood flow, and help prevent injury. Begin gradually, stretching slowly and carefully. Do not bounce or jerk and be careful not to overstretch. When you exercise, start slowly and gradually work up to your target pace.
2. **Aerobic activity of your choice (30 minutes).** You can do this all at once or divide it into two 15-minute sessions or three 10-minute sessions.
3. **Work your muscles (15 minutes).** While your muscles are still warm, strengthen all the muscle groups with simple weight-lifting and toning exercises.
4. **Cool down (10 minutes).** Cooling down after exercise helps prevent muscle soreness and decreases your chances of injury. Be sure to stop exercising slowly and gradually. For example, after jogging, gradually slow down until you are walking, and walk for several minutes. Or, toward the end of a brisk walk, gradually slow your pace. After cooling down, massage your muscles to help your blood circulate. Check your pulse to make sure that it has returned to its normal resting rate.

hour or after work. Or you may prefer to ride a stationary bike or use a treadmill in the privacy of your home while you watch your favorite TV shows. Go over the aerobic activities listed on page 128 and decide which ones seem right for you.

As you can see, there are a number of activities from which to choose, and the list is growing. Today, it is easier than ever to engage in a variety of activities. And variety—which involves choices—is what most people need to keep exercising.

If you like to work out at home by yourself, there are videos for aerobics, flexibility, yoga, and stretching. If you like to work out with other people, you can join a health club or your local

---

WHEN TO STOP EXERCISING

Warning: Never ignore the symptoms of possible overexercise, which could mean that you are having a heart attack or some other medical emergency. Stop exercising **immediately** if you have any of these symptoms:

- Pain or pressure in your chest
- Pain in your neck, jaw, or down your left arm
- Palpitations (a disturbing feeling that your heart is beating irregularly, more strongly, or more rapidly than normal)
- Nausea
- Blurred vision
- Severe shortness of breath
- Faintness or fainting

If you injure yourself, stop exercising immediately. Trying to "work through" the pain could cause more damage to injured tissues. If you have a strain, sprain, or muscle pull, rest the injury for a few days and follow the RICE (rest, ice, compression, and elevation) routine (see page 131). If you think the injury might be serious, talk to your doctor as soon as possible. If you think you have broken a bone, go to your hospital's emergency department.

YMCA or YWCA. Or you can get a friend or a group of friends to join you for walks around a park or at a local shopping mall. Working out with others can help motivate you on days when you are tempted to skip exercise.

If you are physically challenged, you can often find alternative forms of exercise. Ask your doctor what type of exercise is best for you. He or she may refer you to an exercise physiologist, personal

---

RICE ROUTINE FOR FIRST AID

Rest, **i**ce, **c**ompression, and **e**levation—or **RICE**—are the recommended steps for immediate treatment of such minor injuries as sprains, strains, and muscle pulls. If you think your injury might be serious, call your doctor before using RICE.

Rest. Stop exercising and rest the injured part of your body to help reduce swelling and stop further bleeding in the tissues.

Ice. Apply an ice pack to the injured area at regular intervals (about 20 to 30 minutes a session, every 3 hours) over the first several days after an injury. The cold temperature of the ice pack relieves pain and helps limit swelling and bruising by narrowing your blood vessels.

Compression. Place an elastic compression bandage around the injured body part and wear it for at least 2 days. Cover the injured area with the bandage, but also extend it a few inches above and below the injury. Do not wrap the bandage too tightly because it can cut off circulation in the injured part. Loosen the bandage if swelling increases. Like ice, compression helps limit swelling and bruising and relieves pain by supporting injured muscles and tendons.

Warning: If you have diabetes or vascular disease, talk to your doctor before using an elastic bandage; an elastic bandage can interfere with circulation if you wrap it too tightly.

Elevation. When you can, keep the injured part elevated above the level of your heart. Elevation reduces pressure in the tissues, which in turn helps drain any fluids that have collected in the tissues after your injury. Also, elevation reduces swelling and bruising.

---

trainer, or physical therapist for more advice. Swimming and water exercise are sometimes possible. Resistance exercises, in which you tense your muscles but do not move your joints, may be a good choice for you.

Before you begin any exercise regimen, remember that you need to start slowly and increase gradually if you have been inactive. Patience and persistence help you avoid sore muscles and injuries.

HEALTHY EATING

Eating right is an important part of staying healthy. Diet has a tremendous impact on menopausal symptoms and aging-related diseases alike. A good balance of a variety of foods can help prevent a variety of conditions and diseases, from obesity to cardiovascular disease to cancer.

An estimated 67 million Americans, about 1 of 4, now have some form of cardiovascular disease. Several of the leading risk factors for cardiovascular disease, including high cholesterol, obesity, diabetes, and high blood pressure, can all be aggravated by what you eat.

Eating a well-balanced, healthy diet can prolong your life. But deciding which foods are healthy is not easy, especially when you consider that we are often faced with controversial, sometimes even contradictory, nutritional information.

The best diet for a woman approaching menopause and middle age is one in which vegetables, whole grains, fruit, and foods high in calcium take center stage. Such a diet can supply plenty of nutrients without causing obesity or heart disease or other ill effects. Meats should play a lesser role because of their high fat content. And other foods high in fat, sugar, salt, and calories should be used minimally, if at all.

When you make the switch to a healthier diet, you may notice that some health problems slowly lessen. Your energy and endurance level will increase, your weight will stabilize, your hair will look healthier and may stop falling out, your skin may look and feel better, and any problems with constipation should improve.

The Food Guide Pyramid

To help people better follow a healthy diet, the US Department of Agriculture (USDA) developed the Food Guide Pyramid. The USDA recommends that about 60 percent of our calories come from carbohydrates, 30 percent from fat, and 10 percent from protein. The Food Guide Pyramid translated these percentages into servings of specific kinds of food.

The Food Guide Pyramid is designed to help people better understand what foods they need, from what groups, and in what amounts. The main difference between the pyramid and the outdated "four basic food groups" is that meat is no longer the most important element in the diet. Instead, rice, pasta, and/or other whole grains, along with fruits and vegetables, should make up the bulk of your diet. Grains, fruits, and vegetables are high in fiber, carbohydrates, and essential vitamins and minerals and generally are low in fat. Meat is still part of a healthy diet, but most people eat much more meat than they need and not nearly enough fruits and vegetables.

The pyramid is based on an average 2,000-calorie-a-day diet. Older women are generally advised to consume about 1,600 calo-

Food Guide Pyramid

A Guide to Daily Food Choices

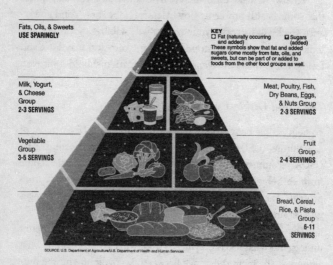

Fats, Oils, & Sweets
USE SPARINGLY

KEY
☐ Fat (naturally occurring and added)   ☑ Sugars (added)
These symbols show that fat and added sugars come mostly from fats, oils, and sweets, but can be part of or added to foods from the other food groups as well.

Milk, Yogurt, & Cheese Group
2-3 SERVINGS

Meat, Poultry, Fish, Dry Beans, Eggs, & Nuts Group
2-3 SERVINGS

Vegetable Group
3-5 SERVINGS

Fruit Group
2-4 SERVINGS

Bread, Cereal, Rice, & Pasta Group
6-11 SERVINGS

SOURCE: U.S. Department of Agriculture/U.S. Department of Health and Human Services

ries a day, depending on their activity level. If you are more active, you may need more calories. On the basis of a 1,600-calorie-a-day diet, it is recommended that you consume six servings of bread, cereal, rice, or pasta, three servings of vegetables, two servings of fruit, two to three servings of low-fat dairy products (milk, yogurt, cottage cheese), and two servings of meat, poultry, fish, or beans. Serving sizes are small to help you stay within this calorie limit. What counts as one serving? **Milk, Yogurt, and Cheese Group:** 1 cup of milk or yogurt; 1½ to 2 ounces of cheese. **Meat,**

Poultry, Fish, Dry Beans, Eggs, and Nuts Group: 2 to 3 ounces of meat, fish, or poultry; ½ cup of cooked dry beans; 1 egg; 2 tablespoons of peanut butter. **Vegetable Group:** 1 cup of raw leafy vegetables; ½ cup of chopped raw or cooked vegetables; ¾ cup of vegetable juice. **Fruit Group:** 1 piece of fresh fruit or melon wedge; ½ cup of canned fruit; ½ cup of dried fruit; ¾ cup of fruit juice. **Bread, Cereal, Rice, and Pasta Group:** 1 slice of bread; 1 ounce of ready-to-eat cereal; ½ cup of cooked cereal, rice, or pasta.

The Food Groups

Take a closer look at the food groups, focusing on those items within each group that have been found to be particularly important to the health of women in midlife.

WHOLE GRAINS

The grain family includes wheat, rye, rice, oats, barley, corn, millet, buckwheat, quinoa, and wild rice. Not only are whole grains good for you, they are delicious. And there are many ways to prepare them. You can eat them whole, as in brown rice; cracked or rolled, as in oatmeal; or ground into whole-grain flours. Grains are a great source of fiber, the indigestible part of plant foods. It is found in different forms in grains, beans, vegetables, and fruits. Fiber helps you fill up naturally, so you are less likely to overeat. In general, it is the fat in the foods we eat that makes us fat.

There are a number of healthy advantages to eating whole grains. Women who eat a diet high in fiber have a lower risk of cancer of the colon and also have fewer problems with gastrointestinal diseases such as diverticulitis. These problems tend to affect women in older age groups. In fact, colon cancer is the third leading cause of cancer and cancer deaths in women. A high-fiber diet also tends to lower blood cholesterol levels, partly by helping metabolize cholesterol and eliminate it from the body more easily. And lower cholesterol levels in the blood decrease the risk of heart attack.

Studies have also shown that a high-fiber, low-fat diet may protect women against breast cancer. Asian and African women consume less fat and three times more fiber than do American women, and these countries have much lower incidences of breast cancer. Vegetarian women in the US, whose diet is lower in fat and higher in fiber, are also reported to have lower breast cancer rates than do meat eaters.

Your goal should be to consume 30 to 35 grams of total fiber each day. The amount of fiber is highest when a food is in its most natural state. Vegetables, fruits, and whole grains will get you the fiber you need. When you increase the fiber in your diet, be sure to drink more water each day, to help prevent constipation.

Here are some tips for getting more whole grains into your diet:

- Buy or make your own whole-grain bread. Skip the added white flour or sugars. Bread machines are making it much easier to bake homemade bread.
- Use brown rice, rolled oats (not instant), rye crackers, fresh corn, corn tortillas, polenta, and buckwheat groats (kasha).
- Start each day with a whole-grain cereal. Read the labels of cereal boxes. If a whole grain is listed, toss that cereal into your shopping cart.

- Use whole-wheat pasta, adding vegetables and low-fat sauces.
- Eat plain popcorn as a snack.

FRUITS AND VEGETABLES

Fruits and vegetables are filled with vitamins and minerals that may help protect against cancer, infections, heart attacks, and stroke. There is evidence that vegetables in the cabbage family— broccoli, brussels sprouts, cabbage, cauliflower, and kale— protect against cancer. These so-called cruciferous vegetables are rich in phytochemicals (plant chemicals) known as indoles, which are the basic components of body substances such as serotonin (a neurotransmitter) and tryptophan (an amino acid). Indoles may trigger the body's production of the enzymes that break down cancer-causing compounds into harmless substances. They appear to be particularly protective against stomach and colon cancers. Broccoli seems to be the most potent vegetable in this family.

Because of their high potassium content, fruits and vegetables are important in a program to reduce blood pressure. Potassium is a mineral similar to sodium. Both are essential to life, but potassium has the opposite effect on blood pressure than sodium does. Evidence suggests that a diet high in potassium and low in sodium tends to bring blood pressure down. Potassium is abundant in winter squashes, beans of all kinds, potatoes, leafy greens, and many fruits, especially bananas.

Here are some suggestions for getting fruits and vegetables into your diet every day:

- Vegetables can be eaten raw or lightly steamed. Water in which vegetables have been cooked can be used as broth,

ANTIOXIDANTS

Antioxidants have received a lot of attention in recent years, and with good reason. Abundant in many fruits and vegetables, antioxidant vitamins—mainly vitamin E, vitamin C, and beta carotene—may decrease the incidence of aging-related diseases such as cancer and heart disease.

In the course of your daily digestion and metabolism, your body uses oxygen, which can form potentially dangerous compounds called free radicals. When not neutralized by antioxidants, free radicals can damage cells and the genes they contain, causing diseases such as cancer and heart disease. Normal body processes, such as breathing and digesting food, produce free radicals. Environmental pollutants, such as cigarette smoke, also produce them.

While the role that free radicals play in disease and aging is not completely understood, some scientists believe they either cause or accelerate the progression of aging-related diseases. Free radicals may cause cancer by damaging deoxyribonucleic acid (DNA). Oxidation of LDL ("bad") cholesterol may be a first step in the development of plaque inside arteries.

Your body has a complex antioxidant system—made up of enzymes, vitamins, and minerals—that neutralizes free radicals before they do their damage. You can obtain antioxidants by eating vegetables, soybeans, and fruits. Whether these self-made and food-derived antioxidants are enough to prevent disease depends on a number of factors, including your overall diet and your lifestyle. By middle age, the body's ability to maintain this antioxidant defense system declines. If levels of free radicals get too high, the body needs even more antioxidant vitamins.

Fruits and vegetables are good sources of antioxidant vitamins. People who eat the most fruits and vegetables have substantially lower cancer rates than those who eat the least. All three antioxidant vitamins—E, C, and beta carotene—appear to affect the formation of blood clots. By reducing the "stickiness" of certain kinds of blood cells, antioxidants make these cells less likely to stick to the inner lining of blood vessels and to each other, thus reducing the chance of potentially life-threatening blood clots.

Below is an in-depth description of each of these vitamins.

Vitamin E. Vitamin E is the primary antioxidant. It also supports the immune system, blocks formation of nitrosamines (suspected cancer-causing substances), and repairs damaged cell membranes. It has been shown to protect against certain types of cancer and heart disease. Vitamin E appears to help fight heart disease by inhibiting the formation of plaque, which can damage the lining of blood vessels. A diet high in vitamin E lowers LDL cholesterol and thus the risk of heart disease. In fact, some studies show that low vitamin E intake is a better predictor of heart disease than elevated cholesterol levels.

Good sources of vitamin E include sunflower seeds, almonds, crab, sweet potatoes, vegetable oils, fish, and wheat germ.

Vitamin C. Vitamin C is believed to defend against cancer in several ways: it deactivates free radicals, it boosts the immune system, it may help fight cancer-causing substances such as pesticides, and may prevent the formation of cancer-causing substances. This vitamin is most strongly associated with protection against gastrointestinal, breast, and cervical cancer.

Vitamin C has also been found to work like vitamin E in preventing heart disease. Vitamin C seems to have an even stronger effect in the oxidation of LDL cholesterol, thus lowering its levels.

Good sources of vitamin C include raw bell peppers, oranges and orange juice, broccoli, cantaloupe, strawberries, fresh tomatoes, and potatoes.

Beta carotene. Beta carotene may help lower the risk of some types of cancer, such as cancer of the lung, breast, cervix, uterus, gastrointestinal tract, and mouth. It also seems to play a role in reducing the risk of heart attack and stroke.

Good sources of beta carotene include spinach, carrots, sweet potatoes, winter squashes, cantaloupe, and broccoli.

because it is high in vitamins, minerals, and the nutrients discussed previously.

- Potatoes and sweet potatoes are excellent vegetables that, contrary to popular belief, do not cause weight gain. Instead, it is the gravy, butter, sour cream, and other toppings that add the fat and calories. Potatoes are best steamed or baked, and can be served with low-fat yogurt or sour cream, low- or nonfat cottage cheese, tomato-based salsa, and chives or other seasonings. They are good sources of protein, vitamin C, and potassium.

- Whenever possible, avoid canned or pickled vegetables, as their sodium content is usually high. Frozen vegetables are a better alternative to canned or pickled vegetables.
- Fruits are best eaten raw, although frozen are much better than canned. Many canned fruits contain added sugar; look for canned fruit packed in fruit juice instead.
- Because fruits are so naturally sweet, you can easily satisfy your sweet tooth with any one of a number of these delicious snacks. Eat fruit for snacks and desserts, instead of chips, ice cream, or pastries.

PROTEIN

Protein is necessary for the growth, maintenance, and repair of every cell in the body. It is present in a number of forms throughout the body—as part of bones, muscle, hair, skin, enzymes, hormones, and antibodies, to name just a few. The body burns carbohydrates for fuel and uses proteins for the building blocks that provide structure and perform vital functions. However, when needed, protein can be broken down to provide energy.

Proteins are composed of many small units called amino acids. Altogether, there are 20 common amino acids. They mix and match in thousands of different combinations to make up specific proteins. The body is unable to make nine of these amino acids, so you must get them from the foods you eat. Proteins in food provide them; the most concentrated sources are red meat, chicken, fish, dairy products, and eggs. Proteins from animal sources are called "complete proteins" because they furnish all the essential amino acids. Most plant proteins—like that found in beans—are incomplete. You can, however, meet your daily protein requirement by eating a variety of plant proteins over the

MOVE OVER, MEAT

To consume a low-fat diet and thereby decrease the risk of heart disease and cancer of the colon, ovary, and breast, try using meat as a flavoring for grains and vegetables rather than as the centerpiece of your meals. For example, cut up lean pieces of meat or fish and stir-fry them with onions, garlic, and vegetables, or make vegetable stews, casseroles, or soups using lean meat as a flavoring.

If you decide to eat less meat, from what foods should you get your daily supply of protein? First, a combination of beans and whole grains or soybeans alone are an excellent source of protein. Dairy products are another excellent protein source. Milk's amino acid balance matches that of meat, fish, and poultry. As with any protein food, dairy products that are lowest in fat are best: nonfat milk, low-fat cottage cheese, low-fat yogurt, buttermilk, kefir, and cheeses such as skim-milk mozzarella and farmer's cheese. (The most popular cheeses—Swiss and cheddar—are highest in fat.) If you replace the meat in your diet with dairy products that are high in fat, you defeat the purpose of avoiding meat.

Some older adults lack the ability to digest milk sugar (lactose) and experience cramping, gas, and diarrhea after drinking milk. This condition is called lactose intolerance. If you are lactose intolerant, sometimes you can eat small servings of cultured milk, such as yogurt, buttermilk, acidophilus milk, and kefir. The milk sugar in these products is partially digested already by bacteria. Also, there are additives available at drugstores that predigest milk sugar and do so without making the milk sour. Soy milk can be used as a milk substitute for drinking, pouring on cereal, and cooking.

If you like meat and do not want to give it up, what should you do? Many doctors agree that people should not eat more than two to three 4-ounce servings of lean meat each day. When you have meat, choose the leanest cuts and trim all visible fat before cooking. Remove and throw away the skin of poultry. Avoid bacon, ham, lunch meat, and pressed or processed meats, as all are high in fat, salt, and chemicals. Frying or broiling meat at a high temperature may produce certain cancer-causing compounds. Use a lower temperature for a longer time or cover the meat and let it simmer slowly.

course of a day. And when you eat plant proteins, you avoid the fat that comes with meat proteins.

Protein supports the cells in muscles, internal organs, blood vessels, skin, and hair. It builds cells during times of growth and repairs them when necessary. But as important as protein is to the maintenance of the body, an excess is not good and may even cause serious problems, such as the following:

- Some meats, especially red meats, are particularly high in saturated fat.
- A high intake of red meats may aggravate premenstrual syndrome (PMS) and menstrual cramps.
- Red meats are high in substances that increase the loss of calcium from the bones, creating a greater risk of osteoporosis.
- Protein may deplete vitamins B_6 and B_3, calcium, and magnesium.
- Processed and smoked meats, such as bacon, ham, salami, and lunch meats, contain nitrates and nitrites, which can lead to the formation of cancer-causing nitrosamines in the body.

Most Americans do not have a problem getting enough protein. In fact, most people get too much protein. Excess protein does not build muscle. It is either burned as energy or stored—not as muscle, but in the form of fat.

Facts on Fat

Fat is important to many body functions. It provides the essential fatty acids needed for normal reproduction and growth as well as

BIG ON BEANS

Beans are an excellent food that is high in protein and fiber and low in fat.

Any bean combined with any grain provides a protein of the same quality as meat, fish, eggs, or milk. For example, a serving of split pea soup with a whole-wheat roll or a serving of black beans with brown rice gives your body protein that is as complete as that in meat.

Another advantage of beans is their high fiber content. The fibrous cover around the bean slows its breakdown in the digestive system, so its nutrients are absorbed into the body more slowly than are other foods. Beans are considered an ideal food for people with diabetes because their slow, regular absorption minimizes the need for insulin.

If intestinal gas bothers you when you eat beans, you can take steps to avoid the problem. Begin with dry beans. Cover them with plenty of water and let them soak for 12 hours or overnight. Throw away the soaking water, rinse the beans, and cook them in fresh water. This process reduces the starches that cause intestinal gas. Also try fresh or frozen beans and peas, bean sprouts, and soybean foods, such as tofu. These do not tend to cause gas.

---

for the production of substances that help regulate blood pressure, blood clotting, and inflammation. Fat cushions bones and vital organs, protects the body from extreme temperatures, carries fat-soluble nutrients, and serves as an important energy reserve.

What makes up a high-fat diet? And what should your fat intake be? Most dietitians agree that you should aim for no more than 30 percent of your daily calories from fat. Where that fat comes from also matters, since certain types of fat are more likely to raise blood cholesterol, which is associated with an increased incidence of atherosclerosis.

Fat contains 9 calories per gram; carbohydrates and protein contain 4 calories per gram each. When you eat carbohydrates—

PROTEIN FROM PLANTS

Whole-grain products	Sunflower seeds	Almonds
Dried beans	Chickpeas	Tofu
Pasta	Cornmeal	Bulgur products
Pecans	Peanuts	Oats
Lentils	Walnuts	Cashews
Barley	Dried peas	Lima beans
Sesame seeds	Rice	

potatoes, rice, pasta, bread, fruits, and vegetables—most are converted to body heat and glycogen. Glycogen is stored in the muscles and liver and serves as a source of energy throughout the day. The fat you eat is mainly stored as fat.

TYPES OF FAT

There are three types of fat: polyunsaturated, monounsaturated, and saturated. Saturation refers to the chemical structure of a particular fat. In general, the more saturated a fat is, the more solid it is at room temperature.

Polyunsaturated fats. Polyunsaturated fats are liquid at room temperature. They are found in plant oils, including sunflower, safflower, soybean, sesame seed, and corn oils. They also appear in fish such as tuna, salmon, and mackerel. Polyunsaturated fats help lower blood cholesterol levels and, when found in fish oils, may act as a blood thinner, decreasing the risk of life-threatening blood clots. These fats still have calories, however, and should be consumed in limited amounts. Ten percent of your total calories should come from polyunsaturated fats.

IN THE SWIM WITH FISH

Some types of fish have a protective effect against heart disease, because of the special kind of fat it contains. The oil in fish has been shown to lower blood levels of cholesterol and to counteract the tendency of blood to clot. Nutritionists often suggest that women include fish in their diets once a week, emphasizing cold-water fish, such as salmon, mackerel, trout, and herring.

The beneficial fat found in fish, known as omega-3 fatty acid or alpha-linolenic acid, is found in few plant foods, with the exception of flaxseed. You can purchase fish-oil supplements over the counter in most drugstores. Some people find that skin problems and painful joints are helped by adding omega-3 fatty acids to their diets.

Monounsaturated fats. Monounsaturated fats are found in fish oils, as well as in olive oil, peanut oil, canola oil, and avocado. If you substitute monounsaturated fat for saturated fat in your diet, it may possibly lower your cholesterol level. The recommended range of monounsaturated fats is no more than 10 percent to 15 percent of total calories. However, you should not use large amounts of monounsaturated oils. They contain some saturated fats and are high in calories. It is best to use only small amounts of fat of any kind.

Saturated fats. Saturated fats are easy to identify because they are usually solid at room temperature. They are found most often in foods that come from animal sources, such as meat and whole-fat dairy products. Some vegetable fats—palm oil and coconut oil, in particular—are also saturated. The more saturated fat you eat, the greater your chances of developing coronary artery disease. Saturated fats may actually raise blood cholesterol levels more than dietary cholesterol does.

THE EGG CONTROVERSY

Eggs are a high-protein food. They are low in fat and high in iron. Because of the high cholesterol content of egg yolks, however, most people should consume them in moderation (three or four a week). And you should avoid yolks completely if you have an elevated cholesterol level or any problem involving blocked arteries in the heart, brain, or legs. When you do eat eggs, it is much healthier to eat them poached, boiled, or baked in food rather than fried in fat. If you want to limit your fat and cholesterol intake, use egg whites and avoid the yolks. Make an omelet with one whole egg and two egg whites, for example, or use commercially available egg substitutes that do not contain cholesterol.

Another form of saturated fat is hydrogenated vegetable oil. Manufacturers take an unsaturated fat, such as soybean oil, and solidify it through a process called hydrogenation. The result is a product such as margarine. Hydrogenated vegetable fats have less saturated fat than butter, but they are not better for you. They still have an unfavorable effect on cholesterol level and have been linked to heart disease. Partially hydrogenated vegetable oils are found in many candies, cakes, pastries, cookies, crackers, and potato chips. Read food labels carefully and avoid those foods with saturated fats listed in their ingredients.

CUTTING THE FAT

Fats in the form of butter, margarine, oil, mayonnaise, cream, and lard are high in calories and low in nutrients. The average American woman consumes about 35 percent of her daily calories in fat; 30 percent or less is recommended. A high-fat diet has been strongly linked to heart disease, stroke, and various cancers, especially cancer of the breast, ovary, and colon. Because these diseases account for more than half the deaths in the US, you are urged to change your eating habits, with the goal of moving toward a low-fat diet. You can do this without major disruption, if you have the right attitude and devise a realistic eating plan.

Here are some suggestions for cutting the fat in your diet:

• Use high-fat dairy products, such as butter, sour cream, ice cream, whipped cream, half-and-half, and whole milk sparingly. About 75 percent of the calories in hard cheeses of all kinds are fat; hard cheeses should be used in small amounts for flavor. Low-fat cottage cheese, low-fat and nonfat yogurt, and nonfat milk are good alternatives and are useful in cooking as well.

• Most people want some fat for better taste; try eating bread or potatoes with a little olive oil and garlic rather than butter or margarine. Use low-fat, low-sodium chicken broth in place of butter in mashed potatoes. Use just a little oil in frying and avoid deep-fried foods. Grill, roast, bake, barbecue, broil, stir-fry, microwave, or poach foods without added fat. Use nonstick pans or nonstick spray. Sauté food in broth or water instead of oil. Make salad dressings with more lemon, vinegar, spices, and low-fat yogurt and less oil or mayonnaise. Cut down by a third or more on the fat required in recipes. Buy a cookbook with low-fat recipes, borrow one from the library, or subscribe to a cooking magazine that features low-fat recipes.

• Eat seeds and nuts sparingly. They can be healthy but have a high fat content. Walnuts and almonds, without added salt or oil, have been found to lower cholesterol levels.

• Avoid ice cream. Fat-free frozen yogurt or fruit sorbet as an occasional treat are much healthier options.

• Choose lean cuts of red meat, such as beef round.

• Snack on low-fat pretzels, plain popcorn, rice or corn cakes, animal crackers, fruits and vegetables, or whole-grain dry cereal.

• Read food labels. Ingredients are listed according to quantity, from the highest to the lowest. Check the amounts of total fat and saturated fats "per serving," as serving size may be smaller than you think. Be sure you are eating just one serving.

• Make healthful choices while dining out. It is not as hard as it used to be to find low-fat foods on most menus. Avoid restaurant food that is rich in butter, oil, cheese, and sauces. The conscientious diner can find steamed or broiled fish without added butter, salad or baked potatoes with dressing on the side, and similar simple dishes. If you cannot find these choices on the menu, ask your waiter or waitress if your selection can be prepared this way for you.

When you switch to a low-fat diet, you will notice several positive changes. You may feel lighter, more energetic, and less sleepy after meals. You may eat the same volume of food but find it takes longer to eat, because low-fat foods are usually high in fiber and require more chewing, yet you will lose weight more easily and often stabilize at a weight considerably lower than before, without consciously dieting.

Making the switch to a low-fat diet is extremely important for staying well after menopause. It requires know-how and vigilance, but it is very rewarding in terms of energy and resistance to disease. It is best to get into the habit of eating a low-fat diet in childhood, but it is never too late to start. The risk of heart disease increases after menopause, making a low-fat diet—along with a regular exercise program—more important than ever.

Cholesterol

Cholesterol, like fat, is essential to the body. But, unlike fat, the liver produces all the cholesterol the body needs; you do not need any additional cholesterol in your diet. Nevertheless, most Americans get plenty of it. Many foods contain cholesterol—some much more than others. Because cholesterol is made by the liver, only animal products contain cholesterol. It is not a component of peanut butter, margarine, or vegetable oils. It is most abundant in eggs and organ meats (such as liver), but some is found in all animal products.

Some people seem more sensitive to high intakes of dietary cholesterol than others. For everyone, however, dietitians recommend an intake of no more than 300 milligrams of cholesterol per day. You can do a lot to achieve a healthier cholesterol level by controlling your diet. Reducing cholesterol and fat intake, particularly saturated fats, will lower total cholesterol levels. Monounsaturated fatty acids (olive and canola oil) tend to raise HDL ("good") cholesterol, so those are the healthiest oils to choose for cooking. Polyunsaturated oils (safflower, corn) lower LDL ("bad") cholesterol, which is good, but they also lower HDL cholesterol, which is not so good. The worst offenders are the saturated fats (meat fat, butter), which raise LDL cholesterol and lower HDL cholesterol.

Vitamins and Minerals

Vitamins regulate crucial functions within the cells of the body. Though needed in only small amounts, they play an important role in storage and production of energy, and they help in tissue formation.

There are 13 essential vitamins. They are classified as either water soluble or fat soluble, depending on how they are transported and stored within the body. This distinction is important. Because the water component of the body turns over frequently, you have to replenish water-soluble vitamins daily. Fat-soluble vitamins are stored in your body fat. This means that you do not need to consume them on a daily basis, and also that taking excessive amounts may lead to levels that are too high.

Vitamin C and the B-complex vitamins are part of the water-soluble group of vitamins. Vitamin A, D, and E are fat-soluble vitamins.

Like vitamins, minerals are necessary for certain functions in the body. They regulate processes such as nerve transmission, blood clotting, and oxygen transport. Most important, minerals provide the framework of the body, or bones. There are 60 minerals in the body, but seven are primary: calcium, phosphorus, magnesium, potassium, sodium, chlorine, and sulfur. All others, needed in tiny amounts, are called trace minerals. Quantity does not necessarily indicate importance, however. Iron, for example, is needed in only trace amounts but is involved in one of the body's most important functions—the transport of oxygen in red blood cells.

Women of all ages need to consume four key minerals to maintain health: calcium, iron, potassium, and sodium.

VITAMINS AND MINERALS FOR MIDLIFE

Here is a list of the vitamins and minerals most important to health in midlife.

Vitamin C. The antioxidant vitamin C enhances the immune system, strengthens bone and blood vessels, aids in iron absorption, and promotes wound healing. The recommended daily allowance (RDA), as determined by the USDA, for vitamin C is 60 milligrams—100 milligrams if you are a smoker (smokers have lower blood levels of vitamin C than nonsmokers). From 4 to 8 ounces of orange juice will supply this amount. Other good sources include citrus fruits, strawberries, cantaloupe, tomatoes, broccoli, potatoes, sweet potatoes, and greens.

Niacin (B_3), thiamin (B_1), and riboflavin (B_2). The B vitamins niacin, thiamin, and riboflavin are important in the processes that produce energy from nutrients. The RDA for niacin is 19 milligrams; for thiamin, it is 1.4 milligrams; and for riboflavin, it is 1.2 milligrams. These vitamins are widely available in low-fat dairy products, meats, fish, poultry, whole-grain breads and cereals, and nuts. Larger doses of niacin (about 100 milligrams) are sometimes prescribed by doctors for the vitamin's cholesterol-lowering properties. However, high doses can cause problems for people with chronic liver disease, gallbladder disease, or peptic ulcer. Common side effects include flushing and gastrointestinal upset.

Folic acid. Another B vitamin, folic acid (or folate), is required for the formation of all new cells. Along with vitamin B_{12}, it is involved in the production of red blood cells. A deficiency of either of these vitamins can cause anemia, fatigue, and slowed mental ability. Because folic acid is involved in creating normal red blood cells, a deficiency causes fewer cells to be produced, which eventually leads to less oxygen making it to all the cells. It is recommended that all women of reproductive age take 400 micrograms (0.4 milligrams) of folic acid daily as a supplement, to reduce the risk of birth defects that can occur during the first 3 months of pregnancy, before many women even know they are pregnant. Folic acid deficiency is common in women, especially older women. Folic acid and vitamin B_{12} work together and so are best consumed that way.

The RDA for vitamin B_{12} is 2 micrograms. It is found only in animal products: meat, fish, poultry, eggs, and dairy products. The RDA for folic acid is 200 micrograms. Folic acid is most plentiful in liver, leafy green vegetables, beans, and seeds; it is also found in whole grains.

Vitamin B_6. Vitamin B_6 is involved in red blood cell formation, the release of glucose (sugar) from storage, and conversion of the amino acid tryptophan into niacin. Vitamin B_6 levels are often low in women.

The RDA for vitamin B_6 is 2 milligrams. Good sources include bananas, avocados, cheese, fish, potatoes, and spinach.

Vitamin A. Vitamin A plays a role in vision, immune and stress responses, energy production, blood production, maintenance of the nervous system and other body tissues, and normal growth and reproduction. Vitamin A deficiency affects the ability of the skin and linings of internal organs to resist cancer, particularly of the skin, lung, bladder, and pharynx.

The RDA for vitamin A is 5,000 international units. It is found in butter, eggs, cheese, fortified low-fat milk, cream, fortified margarine, broccoli, greens, and liver. Another good source of vitamin A is foods rich in beta carotene. In your body, the beta carotene in the foods you eat is converted to vitamin A. Beta carotene is a bright orange color, and it is found in apricots, cantaloupes, squash, carrots, and sweet potatoes.

Vitamin D. Like calcium, vitamin D is critical to maintaining healthy bones. It helps maintain blood calcium levels by regulating the absorption of calcium from the digestive system and its excretion in the urine. An increased intake of vitamin D improves calcium absorption in women of all ages and people with osteoporosis.

The RDA for vitamin D is 400 international units. The best sources are butter, fortified low-fat milk, fortified margarine, eggs, and liver. It is also produced in the intestinal tract by bacteria and is manufactured by skin exposed to sunlight. The average person needs only 10 to 15 minutes in the sun each day to make enough vitamin D. Keep in mind, however, that sunscreens block vitamin D synthesis. However, this is no reason to avoid using sunscreen, as the risk of skin cancer is greater than the risk of getting insufficient amounts of sunlight to manufacture your own vitamin D. Your best bet is to get the vitamin D you need from the foods you eat or from a vitamin supplement.

Vitamin E. An antioxidant, vitamin E is important to the lungs and red blood cell membranes. It also protects white blood cells, which play a major role in the immune system's defense against disease.

The RDA for vitamin E is 25 international units. The leading sources are polyunsaturated vegetable oils, green leafy vegetables, wheat germ, whole grains, nuts, and seeds.

Vitamin K. Vitamin K helps blood to clot. Without vitamin K, wounds would bleed for long periods of time and surgery would be impossible. Bacteria in the intestine can make vitamin K, and because of this, deficiencies do not normally occur. Vitamin K is found in green leafy vegetables and liver. The RDA for vitamin K is 70 milligrams.

Calcium. As discussed earlier, most women do not get enough calcium. Most of the calcium in the body is stored in bones and teeth. Calcium is deposited and withdrawn from bones

GOOD SOURCES OF CALCIUM

FOOD	SERVING	CALCIUM (milligrams)
1% low-fat milk	1 cup	350
Calcium-fortified orange juice	1 cup	320
Low-fat yogurt	1 cup	300
Collard greens, cooked	½ cup	180
Salmon, canned with bones	3 ounces	170
Spinach, cooked	½ cup	140
Calcium-fortified tofu	4 ounces	150
Low-fat cottage cheese	1 cup	120
Corn tortilla	2	120
Great northern beans	½ cup	105
Kale, cooked	½ cup	100

throughout life. In childhood and adolescence, more calcium is deposited than taken out. Later in life, the opposite is true. Calcium levels in the blood must remain within a certain range in order to maintain healthy bones.

One major risk factor for osteoporosis is consistently low calcium intake. Failure to consume enough calcium early in life will result in a failure to form optimally dense bone as an adult, and then you will have less bone to spare as you get older. Bone loss is greatest for the first 5 to 10 years after menopause because of a decline in estrogen. Prior to menopause, estrogen helps to maintain bone density.

The current recommendation for calcium consumption from the National Institutes of Health (NIH) is 1,000 to 1,500 milligrams for most women (1,000 milligrams if taking hormone replacement therapy [HRT]; 1,500 milligrams if not taking HRT or if over age 65). By far, the most concentrated sources of calcium are low-fat milk and dairy products. There are smaller amounts in dark green leafy vegetables, broccoli, calcium-processed tofu, sardines, salmon (including bones), and some fortified cereals (see Good Sources of Calcium, page 154).

In addition to its benefits for bone, calcium also seems to have a positive effect on high blood pressure in some people. Exactly how this works has not yet been determined. But it is another good reason for making sure you get at least the recommended amount of calcium each day.

Because most women get only about 500 milligrams of calcium per day from their diet, many doctors recommend taking calcium supplements to bring the total amount up to the recommended level. Also, many women have lactose intolerance, and eating dairy products may cause painful bloating, gas, and diarrhea. For these reasons, you may want to consider taking calcium supplements. Ask your doctor for a recommendation.

Iron. The mineral iron plays an important role in the transport of oxygen throughout the body. It also helps the body use

GOOD SOURCES OF IRON

FOOD	SERVING	IRON (milligrams)
Oatmeal	¾ cup	8.35
Spinach, cooked	I cup	6.4
Kidney beans	I cup	5.3
Iron-fortified cereal	I½ cups	4.5
Sirloin steak	3 ounces	3.4
Raisins	⅔ cup	2.08

beta carotene and clears fats from the blood. Most iron in the body is stored in hemoglobin, a protein that transports oxygen from the lungs to the tissues in red blood cells.

Many women do not get enough iron. They do not consume enough iron-rich foods, and the iron in the foods they eat is not used completely by the body. An inadequate intake of iron, excessive bleeding, or heavy menstrual periods can cause iron-deficiency anemia. This form of anemia is characterized by a reduction in the number of red blood cells and the amount of hemoglobin in the blood. A deficiency of hemoglobin reduces the amount of oxygen delivered to cells. Symptoms of anemia include fatigue and lowered resistance to infections.

It can be difficult to get enough iron from your diet. The RDA for iron is 18 milligrams. Even if you make an effort to eat the required amount of iron-rich foods each day, you still have to take into account the fact that the body does not absorb dietary iron completely. Only about 10 percent of the iron ingested is actually used by the body. Some women will benefit from taking an iron supplement, particularly if they do not eat red meat regularly.

Good sources of iron include lean red meat, liver, dried apricots, blackstrap molasses, raisins, beans, cooked spinach, chicken, and iron-fortified cereals. Certain chemicals used in the production and packaging of foods diminish the body's ability to absorb iron. Tannic acid (found in many teas), phytic acids (an ingredient in grains and cereals), and phosphates (a preservative added to many packaged foods) greatly decrease the body's use of iron. Look for these ingredients on food labels if you are concerned about your iron intake. On the other hand, vitamin C aids in the absorption of iron, so be sure to get plenty of vitamin C.

Potassium. The mineral potassium is needed for muscles to contract properly, for nerve transmission, and for proper functioning of the heart and kidneys. It also helps to maintain fluid balance in the cells. In addition, some studies indicate that potassium may lower blood pressure in certain individuals.

Most potassium is absorbed in the digestive tract, and the kidneys regulate how much potassium is in the blood by resorbing what is needed and excreting the excess in the urine.

Potassium deficiency is rare. However, people with high blood pressure who take a diuretic need to be sure they get enough potassium in their diet. Diuretics flush excess water out of the body, and potassium goes along with it.

Although there is no established RDA for potassium, the minimum requirement is estimated to be 1,600 to 2,000 milligrams per day. The best sources of potassium are oranges, orange juice, bananas, potatoes, dried fruits, yogurt, milk, meat, and poultry.

Sodium. The sodium in table salt (sodium chloride) and many packaged foods can contribute to high blood pressure and osteoporosis. Research has also shown that the chloride portion of table salt may also raise blood pressure.

Americans tend to oversalt their foods. Not everyone develops blood-pressure problems related to sodium intake, but certain people are salt sensitive. Genetics appears to play a role, because people with a family history of high blood pressure are more likely to develop the problem if they salt their foods. African Americans seem to be especially at risk for high blood pressure—possibly due to a genetic sensitivity to salt intake.

Most people should limit their salt intake. This is pretty easy to do. Here are some ideas:

- Cook with little or no added salt. Use other flavorings in its place, such as onions, garlic, lemon juice, herbs, and spices. A little experimentation will help you find tasty alternatives.
- Avoid processed foods, such as canned soups and vegetables, pickles, olives, salted nuts, potato chips, soy sauce, and hard cheeses.
- When dining out, request that the kitchen go easy on the salt. Restaurant food can be oversalted. Order Chinese food without monosodium glutamate (MSG).
- Taste food before adding salt.
- If you have difficulty becoming accustomed to the taste of unsalted food, wean yourself gradually. Salt is an acquired taste. Children brought up without it grow into adults who do not crave it, and adults can gradually condition themselves to enjoy food with less added salt. Start by adding half the amount of salt that you normally would. Then add only a quarter. Soon you will realize that food tastes better without any added salt.

While high blood pressure has been treated successfully for years with drugs, antihypertensive medications may have unpleasant side effects, such as fatigue, dizziness, or decreased sex drive. Many people with mild hypertension can successfully bring down their blood pressure merely by lowering their salt and fat intake; losing excess weight; avoiding alcohol; quitting smoking; eating plenty of vegetables, fruits, and calcium; exercising regularly; and using relaxation techniques (see page 177).

There is no RDA for sodium. Most healthy people should not consume more than 2,400 milligrams of sodium per day. Food labels include the amount of sodium per serving to help you evaluate your daily intake. You may be amazed at how much sodium you consume in just one serving of a packaged food product, such as canned soup or potato chips.

SHOULD YOU TAKE A SUPPLEMENT?

The best way to get the vitamins and minerals you need is by eating a well-balanced, varied diet. While individual vitamins and minerals are essential to good health, it may be the combination of these and other essential nutrients in the foods we eat that really keeps our bodies functioning well. Vitamins and minerals need fiber, water, and carbohydrates to do their best work. It is for this reason that food is still the best source of vitamins and minerals.

However, every woman has days, weeks, months, and even years in which she just cannot seem to get enough of certain vitamins or minerals. You are most likely to be missing some vitamins or minerals if you smoke, are dieting, are recovering from surgery or an illness, have heavy menstrual bleeding, are vegetarian, have digestive problems, or are under stress. Then it may be a good idea for you to take a multivitamin-multimineral supplement.

In general, vitamin and mineral supplements can be useful as long as the amounts of certain vitamins, such as A and D, are not too high and the doses of minerals are close to the RDA. Too much of these vitamins and minerals can be toxic and cause ill effects.

People with specific diseases and conditions may need a supplement to make up for deficiencies caused by their health problems. This includes those who are malnourished, those with impaired digestion, those on medications that block the body's use of a certain nutrient, those with extra nutritional requirements, vegetarians, women with heavy vaginal bleeding, and women at risk of osteoporosis. If you fall into one of these groups or decide you want a supplement to improve your overall health, talk with your doctor.

Water

Water is often left off the list of nutrients that make up a healthy diet. And yet, next to oxygen, it is the most important nutrient. A healthy adult can survive for weeks without food but only days without water.

Water is the major component of body fluid, making up a little more than half of the body weight of an average adult female. Water plays a major role in the body, demonstrated by the fact that it:

- Is crucial to the formation of blood
- Flushes wastes from the body
- Keeps the kidneys and sweat glands functioning properly
- Keeps food moving through the digestive system
- Facilitates the transportation of nutrients and hormones to the cells
- Regulates body temperature by bringing heat to the skin surface in the form of sweat, thus cooling the body and preventing heat stroke or other heat-related illnesses
- Is a source of minerals that are important to the blood, bones, and heart

As you age, your body loses about 10 percent to 15 percent of its fluid. Dehydration becomes more common as you get older.

The signs of dehydration include lethargy, muscle weakness, and constipation.

You get some water from the foods you eat, but most of it comes from consuming fluids such as juice, milk, soup, and water. Ideally, you should drink six to eight 8-ounce glasses of water every day.

Sugar

Simple white sugar (sucrose) and its variations, such as fructose, are added to many packaged foods, including cakes, cookies, soft drinks, ice cream, candy, cold cereals, and others. Honey, maple sugar, and molasses are added to many health-food products. All forms of sugar provide empty calories (calories without nutrients).

For optimum health, eat sparingly foods that contain added sugar. Instead, satisfy cravings for sweets with fresh and dried fruits, such as prunes, raisins, figs, and dates. The sugar you get in fruit is supplemented by vitamins, potassium, and other minerals. Also, fruit has fiber but no added fat or salt. People who eat fruit and avoid refined sugar have far less tooth decay.

Many people use sugar substitutes, such as aspartame and saccharin, in desserts, soft drinks, and coffee. Very large doses of saccharin cause bladder cancer in some experimental animals. The US Food and Drug Administration (FDA) requires a warning label about cancer on products that contain saccharin. Aspartame is another sugar substitute that appears in many soft drinks and packaged products. It cannot be used by people with phenylketonuria (PKU), a condition in which the body cannot metabolize aspartame. For everyone else, however, aspartame is a safe, useful way of avoiding excess calories from sugar.

Caffeine

Caffeine is a drug that stimulates the central nervous system, making you feel more energetic. As a diuretic, it increases the blood flow through your kidneys, which produce more urine as a result. Coffee, tea, cola drinks, chocolate, some pain relievers, and many over-the-counter energy aids contain caffeine.

Large amounts of caffeine cause you to lose more calcium in your urine, which is a risk factor for osteoporosis. Also, caffeine can aggravate premenstrual breast tenderness in some women. Caffeine can cause nervousness or a jittery feeling, and you should avoid caffeine if it triggers hot flashes.

Putting It All Together

Always keep in mind that the way you eat now can make a big difference later in your quality of life. It is a good idea to focus on eating foods that will help prevent aging-related diseases such as heart disease, cancer, and osteoporosis. You cannot go wrong with a high-fiber, low-fat diet, a diet naturally rich in fruits and vegetables, whole grains, and low-fat dairy products. Such a diet not only is good for the long term but also makes you feel better from day to day.

While some weight gain with age may be normal, there is much you can do to stay trim. Limit your fat intake to less than 30 percent of your daily calories. Cutting back on fat is the easiest way of holding down your total caloric intake each day. Remember, too, that your bones depend on a consistent intake of calcium and vitamin D, particularly after menopause. And given all the known and assumed health benefits of fruits and vegetables, make

TEN STEPS TO A HEALTHIER DIET

To sum it all up, here are 10 steps you can take to keep your diet on the right track:

1. Pinpoint sources of fat. Your goal is to keep total fat calories below 30 percent, on average.
2. Keep your cholesterol intake to less than 300 milligrams per day.
3. Eat five or more servings of fruits and vegetables each day. In general, a serving is one small piece of fruit, ½ cup of cooked vegetables, or 1 cup of raw vegetables. Fruits and vegetables are high in antioxidants and fiber.
4. Increase your intake of complex carbohydrates, especially whole grains.
5. Watch your protein intake. Most women need only about 6 ounces of meat, chicken, or fish per day.
6. Drink alcohol only in moderation. Excessive drinking is linked to osteoporosis and may cause falls, leading to fractures.
7. Limit daily salt intake to 2,400 milligrams; even less is better.
8. Eat a high-calcium diet or take calcium supplements.
9. Take a multivitamin-multimineral supplement that contains iron if you do not get enough of these important nutrients in your diet.
10. Drink six to eight glasses of water, at least 8 ounces each, every day.

every effort to include them as a major part of your diet—at least three to five servings of vegetables and two to four servings of fruit each day.

Whether you are 40, 60, or 80, the current RDAs are the same, but individual needs may vary. Health problems may make it necessary for you to increase certain nutrients or cut back on or avoid others. Talk to your doctor if you have questions about your diet.

As they get older, some people may find that they tend to eat less. Chewing problems, digestive disorders, or even having to eat alone all may contribute to this. If this is the case, you need to make every meal count, by eating a highly nutritious, well-balanced diet. You should eat as much fiber as possible to keep your colon healthy and avoid constipation, plenty of calcium-containing foods to help prevent osteoporosis, and perhaps some extra iron, if your doctor thinks it is necessary. If you find that it is impossible to maintain a balanced diet, you may need to take a multivitamin with minerals. Talk to your doctor before taking vitamins or supplements.

As you work on your diet, keep a few things in mind. First, you are looking to strike a balance. If you splurge and have more high-fat foods one day, compensate by lowering your fat intake over the next couple of days. Not every food you eat will have the recommended percentage of fat, protein, carbohydrates, and so on. Your goal is to get what is recommended over the course of a day or maybe even a week. Second, there are no good or bad foods, only those that should be eaten more or less often, and those for which you should control your portion sizes more carefully. If your usual diet is rich in carbohydrates and low in fat, an occasional celebration will do you no harm. While you focus on cutting back on fat, increase your intake of health-protecting fruits, vegetables, and whole grains. Think of healthy eating as a lifestyle choice, not a diet. The changes you make should be manageable enough to last your lifetime.

MANAGING STRESS

Stress, at any age, is an inevitable part of life. At menopause, it is a natural consequence of change, both because of physical changes and the attitudes that people bring to the situation. But while menopausal mood swings do occur, not all women get them and they are not always uncontrollable. Chances are good that if you have had mood swings just before your periods, you will probably experience mood swings during perimenopause.

If you already know how to manage stress, you will not lose this ability with menopause. And if you are not very good at handling stress, there is a lot you can learn. After all, you cannot escape stress, but you can change how you cope with it.

What Is Stress?

Stress is a physical and psychological response to a disruption of your usual sense of well-being. Stress causes tension and an increased sense of alertness. Stressors are situations that require you either to adapt or to face the consequences. Any significant change in your routine, positive or negative, can cause stress. Retirement, for example, is a stressor that requires you to make changes: you must adjust financially and you have to find new ways to spend your time. Not all stressors are negative. For some, retirement is a welcome event; for others, the thought of having no job is extremely stressful. Getting a promotion, becoming a grandparent, buying a new house, and other positive events are stressors because they require life-changing adjustments.

Stress and Health

When faced with a stressor, your body responds with a chain of reactions that affects your entire system. Any real or imagined emergency sets in motion a series of changes commonly referred to as the fight-or-flight response, so called because the changes are meant to enable the body to fight the "danger" or flee from it. Responding to triggers from the brain, the adrenal glands release adrenaline and other "stress" hormones. These hormones speed up heart rate and breathing, raise blood pressure, dilate pupils, boost blood-sugar levels, and release high-energy fats into the blood to provide the body with quick energy. Overall, you feel a heightened sense of alertness. This stress response was advantageous for people who lived in the hostile environment of long ago who might have had to fight or flee from wild animals and such. But in today's world, this response is not appropriate for the kind of stressors most people encounter, such as traffic jams and arguments. This now needless flooding of the body with stress hormones is why stress has become a suspected cause of the development of a number of illnesses. Unrelieved, unremitting stress keeps your body in a constant state of alertness and can seriously affect your health.

Stress can affect your body's immune response and make you more vulnerable to illness. Studies have shown a relationship between stress and resistance to infection. Doctors are not sure why one person may have abdominal cramping as a result of stress, while another has headaches. Many researchers believe that environmental factors combined with heredity and coping skills determine a person's individual reaction to stressors.

Every person reacts to different stressors in different ways and to different degrees. It is hard to say how much stress is too much. And while positive and negative life events alike are stressful, unpleasant ones take a greater toll on the body, mind, and overall health.

It is really important for you to understand the way your body reacts to stress. That way, you can recognize when stress is becoming too much for you to handle well, and you can initiate steps to manage stress better.

If you experience any of the following symptoms on a frequent basis, it could be that stress is affecting your health.

Heart irregularities. Stress may play a role in the development of heart disease, especially in postmenopausal women. In one study, older women who took stressful mental tests had higher blood pressures and heart rates than did men or younger women. Researchers who monitored members of all three groups as they went about their daily activities noted that postmenopausal women were three times as likely to respond to stress with episodes of abnormal heart function, such as palpitations or irregular heart rhythms. This may be especially dangerous for middle-aged or older women whose arteries are already narrowed and may result in angina (pain in the chest, arm, or jaw caused by lack of oxygen to the heart muscle).

Digestive disorders. The chemical reactions that occur in response to stress have a direct effect on the digestive tract, and women seek medical help for stomach and intestinal problems much more often than men do. There are a number of digestive ailments that have close ties to stress, including ulcers, irritable bowel syndrome, and nonulcer dyspepsia. While irritable bowel syndrome and ulcers are ultimately caused by factors other than stress, being under a lot of stress can aggravate these conditions and make it difficult for your body to overcome them.

If you experience chronic stomach discomfort, talk to your doctor. He or she can investigate the cause and together you can come up with a successful treatment. In the meantime, during times of stress, try not to change your eating habits. Make sure your diet is well balanced and avoid alcohol, caffeine, carbonated beverages, and rich, fried, or fatty foods. In times of stress, it is easy to use these foods as a crutch. Keep a lot of healthy food on hand.

Sleep difficulties. Insomnia is a common problem for women in perimenopause and menopause. It is also one of the most common symptoms of stress. Whether you are under stress from something that is happening in your life or hot flashes and night sweats are not allowing you to get a good night's sleep, insomnia can make a bad situation worse. The less sleep you get, the more stressed you may become. If sleeplessness persists for more than a few days, follow the recommendations for ensuring a good night's sleep outlined on pages 31 through 33.

Fatigue. Fatigue can result from chronic, unrelieved stress; sleep deprivation; or a variety of illnesses. If you feel constant fatigue, first determine whether you are getting all the sleep you need. Sleep restores the body, allowing it to repair damage caused by stress and other factors. Women who lead stressful lives actually need more sleep than do other women, because their bodies demand more sleep recovery time. Sleep-deprived women show diminished mental alertness and performance; over time, unchecked fatigue can lead to depression and illness.

To help fight fatigue, try to determine how much sleep is right for you. Then make a point of getting it regularly. Go to bed a little earlier or take short naps, if possible. Eat a well-balanced diet with plenty of fresh fruits and vegetables and engage in regular exercise—at least 20 to 30 minutes of brisk walking three times a week. Exercise is a great energy booster, no matter what your age.

Migraines and headaches. Migraine and other headaches are frequently due to stress-related factors. Reactions to stress that can trigger headaches include muscle tension in the neck and jaw, teeth grinding, jaw stiffness, and congested sinuses.

A mild to moderate headache will usually respond to over-the-counter pain medication, such as acetaminophen. Avoid products containing aspirin or ibuprofen if you have a sensitive stomach. True migraine headaches—severe pain that causes nausea, diarrhea, and sensitivity to light and keeps you in bed for hours—are more of a challenge. See your doctor if you think you have migraines.

Neck and back pain. When stress produces muscle tension, painful spasms in the neck and back can result. Your posture, the chair you use, the type of work you do, and your muscle tone can affect your susceptibility to back and neck pain.

Hot showers, massages, heating pads, and over-the-counter pain medications are usually enough to relieve simple, temporary back and neck pain. However, preventive measures can help. Include stretching exercises in your daily routine and use a well-designed chair. Learn how to lift and carry heavy objects properly—remember always to bend your knees to lift something off the floor, not your back. And do not be afraid to ask for help in carrying a heavy object.

When back pain is persistent, severe, or incapacitating, see your doctor.

Skin problems. Stress can cause or worsen a wide variety of skin conditions, including acne, hives, eczema, and psoriasis. Because many other factors—including allergies, prescription and over-the-counter medications, and overexposure to the sun—can also affect the skin, the best first step is to seek the advice of your doctor whenever you are troubled with a persistent, uncomfortable rash, eruption, or inflammation.

Emotional problems. Many behavioral and emotional problems, such as anxiety and depression, can be triggered by stress. It is not unusual for stress to make you feel depressed, anxious, or even a little panicky at times. If these feelings cannot be relieved by a healthy diet, exercise, and/or the use of relaxation techniques, if they persist even after the stressful episode has passed, or if they cause serious disruption in your life, it could be a sign of a more serious problem that may require professional help. Do not be afraid to ask for the help you need.

Hair loss. Some women's hair may begin to thin or fall out as they go through menopause. Hair loss can be reduced by taking estrogen as part of HRT. Talk to your doctor if you are concerned about recent hair loss.

Stress and Menopause

Many women experience mood swings in menopause due to hormonal changes, and stress can further aggravate these mood swings. It is understandable that women may react negatively to uncomfortable physiological changes, such as irregular menstrual cycles, vaginal dryness, and insomnia. Normal stress reactions are compounded by internal hormonal changes. The hormonal changes do not actually cause the emotional behavior, but they change the body's equilibrium, turning mild stress into major stress. Menopausal women tend to feel more depressed, anxious, and irritable than premenopausal women. Many women may feel "blue" or angry. However, these feelings should not be dismissed or ignored; they may be warning signs of a serious depression that requires prompt treatment.

There are a number of situations that may cause some women to feel stressed. The so-called empty-nest syndrome, which some women experience as a result of their children's leaving home, was once seen as a major reason for women's menopausal depression. Today, however, most women of this age are leading active and productive lives.

It is interesting to note that a number of women report that a new family situation—which represents the opposite of the empty-nest syndrome—is what is causing their stress. Today, many adult children are moving back home with their parents. Faced with financial hardship and other problems, they have nowhere else to turn. While parents often welcome their children home, it is common for this situation to bring about stress. The young adult children usually want freedom to come and go at all hours, but often they still expect their mothers to wait on them, cook for them, and generally take care of them. And it is the resulting stress that can cause these women, many of whom are menopausal, to become irritable, anxious, and perhaps depressed.

Another problem for many menopausal women today is the "sandwich" phenomenon. Many women of this age find themselves "sandwiched" between taking care of their children and their aging parents. Either these women delayed having children and so still have younger children to raise or their adult children have moved back home. Taking care of children and aging parents, balancing a job outside the home, and also having to deal with the physical symptoms of menopause can be very stressful for women. Again, it is not menopause that causes the mental anguish, but the other demanding life events that can push some women into depression.

If you are experiencing stress as a result of balancing all of your roles—mother, daughter, wife, employee, and so on—it is important that you find time for yourself. This is, of course, easier said than done, but it is vital to your emotional and physical well-being. While you know what your responsibilities to others are, remember that you have an even greater responsibility to yourself. Maintain your sense of emotional balance and be sure to make some time for your own relaxation or pleasure.

While the empty-nest syndrome may not be as common as it once was, some women still experience depression after their children leave home. If this happens to you, you should leave the nest, too. Any activity that boosts your sense of self-worth will take your mind off of the past and onto the future. Find a job or volunteer, go back to school, exercise, socialize; do whatever it takes to get you up and out of the house. Staying active and involved will help your mental health and may also help you fight other symptoms of menopause and prevent the health risks that come with it.

How Stressed Are You?

Before you can take steps to relieve stress, you need to determine the cause. It is difficult to measure stress because each woman has different sources of stress in her life, and what is stressful for one woman may not be stressful for another.

Below are some examples of stressful situations many women in midlife experience. If you are trying to cope with one or more of these, you may be at increased risk of stress-related illness.

Remember that both positive and negative situations can produce stress.

- Death of a spouse
- Death of a close family member or close friend
- Marital problems
- Separation or divorce
- Hospitalization of a family member because of illness
- Retirement (you or your spouse)
- Sexual problems
- Change in financial status (for the better or worse)
- Job change or job loss
- Child leaving or returning home
- A move to a new home
- Problems at work
- Personal illness or injury
- Unwanted or unexpected pregnancy (yours or a child's)

Coping With Stress

Before you can relieve stress, you need to understand how you react to stress. Each woman has her own stress threshold. What is stressful for one woman may not be stressful for another. Recognize your own limits. Know which stressors really get to you. Be aware of the times in your life that are particularly stressful. If you experience a few major stressful events within a short period of time, give yourself some time to adjust. Pamper yourself. Acknowledge that you are going through a difficult time. Try to gain control of the situation by asking yourself, "How can I change this?" Make time to rest and relax. Adopt a program of healthy eating and regular exercise. Or if you are already following such a program, stick with it. Use the coping strategies described below that work best for you. If one does not work so well, try another.

1. **Eat a well-balanced diet.** A well-balanced diet will help you handle stress. But it is very easy to neglect your nutritional needs when you are under a lot of stress. While research has not yet proven a connection between stress and the need for certain vitamins, nutritionists often recommend a diet high in vitamins B, C, and E when stress levels are high. Research on the food–mood connection also suggests that you may be able to relieve some of the anxiety associated with stress by eating a healthy diet.

Here are some other tips for a healthy, stress-fighting diet:

- Eat plenty of raw fruits and vegetables.
- Take in a good amount of complex carbohydrates.
- Eat more fish and poultry.
- Eat a good breakfast every day.
- Avoid high-fat foods.
- Eat foods high in fiber.
- Drink plenty of fluids to relieve stress-related constipation.
- Wait at least 2 hours after dinner before you lie down at night; this helps prevent gastric distress.

2. **Exercise regularly.** Regular exercise is one of the best ways to fight stress. When you exercise, your body produces and releases a group of hormones known as endorphins—the same hormones that produce the "high" experienced by long-distance runners during intensive training. When you have finished a workout, you are left in a state of natural relaxation. Your heart rate decreases and your blood pressure goes down.

To alleviate stress, you should try to engage in some kind of aerobic exercise as often as you can. Exercising twice a day when things are really tough will go a long way toward helping you cope. Try to fit exercise into your daily routine. A 30-minute session is ideal, but you can divide it into two sessions of 15 minutes each, or three sessions of 10 minutes each. Read the section on pages 123 through 132 for more information about starting an exercise program.

3. **Get plenty of rest.** Fatigue can reduce your ability to cope with stress. Do not rely on over-the-counter or prescription sleep medications to break this cycle. Instead, try improving your sleep habits. Read the section on insomnia and how to get a good night's sleep on pages 31 through 33.

4. **Set priorities.** Often, the stressors that affect you most are not major events but are life's everyday annoyances. Try dividing daily tasks into three categories: those that are essential, those that are important, and those that are not necessary. Learn to put aside those tasks that are not necessary. Do not even think about them. Next, delegate as many tasks as you can to coworkers, children, relatives, and your spouse; trying to be a superwoman and doing it all yourself creates more stress. And finally, concentrate on getting the essential tasks done. Be sure to place time for yourself on the top of your list of essentials. Spend a little time each day doing something you enjoy.

5. **Practice relaxation techniques.** There are a number of relaxation techniques designed to reduce stress. Among them are deep breathing, mental imagery, progressive muscle relaxation, yoga, and meditation. The goal of relaxation techniques is to enable you to return to a peaceful, inner calm after periods of stress. They work in two ways. First, they help you to calm down after episodes of anger, fear, or action. Instead of being left with a feel-

ing of emotional turmoil after a stressful episode, you are left feeling calm. And second, they help you to maintain an inner calm most of the time, even during times of stress. Some alternative practitioners recommend deep-breathing techniques and various forms of meditation to help control hot flashes (as opposed to general stress reduction).

Books and videotapes on relaxation methods, meditation, and coping with stress are available from libraries and book and video stores. More information on relaxation techniques is on page 177.

6. **Seek help.** Talking it out may be just what you need to relieve your stress. Support comes in many different forms. The easiest way to seek support is to open up about your stresses and share your feelings with your family, friends, and coworkers. If you have a problem that you feel is too personal to discuss with a close friend or family member, you may want to consider seeking professional help, such as counseling or psychotherapy. Ask your doctor to refer you to a psychologist or psychiatrist. Sometimes, the most sympathetic and helpful listeners are those who share similar problems, so you may want to consider joining a support group. Hospitals, mental-health clinics, and churches and synagogues often sponsor support groups for a variety of emotional concerns, such as divorce or death of a spouse. If you feel overwhelmed by stress, talk to your doctor. He or she will be able to refer you to a qualified therapist or recommend an appropriate support group.

How Not to Cope

It is not uncommon for a person to be tempted to reach for a quick fix in the face of stress. For example, if you smoke, you

RELAXATION TECHNIQUES

Relaxation techniques can help reduce stress. Try these methods and see how they can help you cope.

Meditation. There are a number of ways to meditate. One of the most common methods involves finding a quiet, comfortable place where you can spend 15 to 20 minutes alone in peace. Relax, close your eyes, and try to free your mind of outside thoughts.

Mental imagery. This technique is also known as visualization. It can be used in conjunction with meditation or by itself. Mental imagery can help to calm you down generally or strengthen your body against disease. The theory behind imagery is that if you create strong mental pictures of what you want, while telling yourself that you can and will get it, you can make just about anything happen. It involves imagining changes you want to happen are actually taking place. For example, you might imagine that you are self-confident and better able to deal with stressful situations. After a time, you will become more self-confident, and you will handle stressful situations better. If you are skeptical of mental imagery's effectiveness, bear in mind that it has been found to increase immune function and to help achieve some remarkable cures.

Deep breathing. One of the easiest relaxation techniques to learn is deep breathing. It is also easy to find the time to do it. And you can do it just about anywhere. Deep breathing helps to keep your heart and lungs working efficiently, and it can help to reduce tension. Rapid breathing when you are nervous can lead to hyperventilation, in which it becomes more difficult to breathe.

To perform deep breathing, sit or lie in a comfortable position, close your eyes, and deeply relax all of your muscles. To help you relax, breathe in and out through your nose. For maximum benefit, breathe deeply, pulling air deep into your lungs. When you breathe out, exhale as much air as possible to make room for your next breath. Continue breathing deeply for 10 to 20 minutes.

When you are finished, remain quiet with your eyes closed for a few more moments, then open them gradually.

Progressive relaxation. This technique involves tensing each muscle of the body for a count of 10 and then releasing for a count of 10 before moving on to the next muscle. You generally move through the body in a particular order— either from the extremities inward or from head to toes or toes to head. Enjoy the relaxation interval and try to imagine the blood flow increasing to each set of muscles that you relax.

may take out a cigarette. If you drink, you may turn to alcohol. If you are tired, you may increase your caffeine consumption. In the long run, however, tobacco, alcohol, caffeine, and other drugs only make matters worse. Tobacco intensifies the effects of stress on the nervous system. Nicotine, the active addictive ingredient in cigarettes, promotes the release of epinephrine (a hormone) from the adrenal glands, producing the fight-or-flight reaction within the body. The smoker's heart rate increases, and blood pressure rises.

As for alcohol, you are likely to feel stronger effects from a given amount of alcohol when you are emotionally upset or under stress than you would when drinking the same amount while feeling calm and relaxed.

And while you may be tempted to fight your fatigue during the day by consuming more caffeine, this is not a good idea. Caffeine may actually make you feel more anxious, because its effect on the central nervous system is stronger during times of stress. If you consume caffeine late in the day, it may lead to a vicious circle of nighttime sleeplessness and daytime drowsiness, so cut back on caffeine and find more constructive ways of coping with fatigue. Exercise and relaxation techniques are two good examples of better ways to cope with stress.

Beyond Everyday Stress

If you find that you are feeling stressed beyond what you feel is normal, it may be time to seek professional help. Ask your physician for a referral to a psychiatrist (a physician trained in mental health) or other mental-health professional. Most doctors think that when your negative mood is interfering with your ability to function properly, it is time to seek help. Sometimes individual therapy alone will help. In other cases, medication may be warranted, or both may be needed to restore you to full health. But whatever you do, do not ignore negative emotional symptoms any more than you would ignore chronic physical pain; both can be damaging to your health and your everyday functioning.

8

Menopause and Sexuality

Contrary to what many people think, women can enjoy an active and fulfilling sex life throughout their menopausal years. While some physical responses slow with age, the capacity and need for sexual expression continues. Naturally, health problems tend to become more common in the menopausal years. But while many of these problems may impact sexual activity and increase the occurrence of sexual problems, there is no reason why women cannot have fulfilling sex lives after age 50. While it seems that menopause either contributes to or coincides with some decrease in sexual desire, not everyone experiences that, and not everyone who does considers it a problem. It appears that treatable menopausal symptoms—vaginal dryness, hot flashes, and so on—rather than menopause itself, contribute to sexual problems. There is no solid evidence that lower estrogen levels are a direct cause of decreased interest in sex.

If you want an active sex life, you may need to work at it. Know what to expect of yourself and your partner, keep the lines of communication open, and be open to new alternatives. Be aware that both you and your partner are going through physical changes that may affect your sexual relationship. With knowledge, patience, and, in some cases, medical treatment, you can help ensure that you will be sexually active for the rest of your life.

PHYSICAL CHANGES THAT AFFECT SEX

As discussed earlier, menopause causes physical changes in the female reproductive organs and affects hormonal secretions. Some of these changes may result in a temporary decline in sexual responsiveness. Fluctuating hormone levels at this time of life account for many unpleasant symptoms, including hot flashes, fatigue, and mood swings, which may make you feel generally unwell. If you experience hot flashes, headaches, and night sweats, for example, you may not feel like engaging in sexual activity. But for many women who lose interest in sex, the cause has more to do with symptoms such as vaginal dryness, which can lead to painful intercourse.

This is a review of the specific physical changes that take place at menopause that may contribute to a loss of sexual desire:

• The vagina becomes dryer, narrower, and less elastic. Estrogen nourishes the vaginal lining, and once the hormone is depleted, this effect diminishes. Without estrogen stimulation, the vaginal lining loses its tough outer layer of protective cells and becomes thinner, smoother, less elastic, and more easily traumatized. Already-sensitive tissues may become inflamed and irritated with sexual intercourse. All of these symptoms can interfere with your ability to enjoy sex. And the tendency for vaginal narrowing and shortening tends to increase if a woman does not have regular intercourse.

- As estrogen levels fall, blood flow to the genitals diminishes and secretions of vaginal lubrication decrease. A woman generally is slower to lubricate in response to sexual arousal and often takes a little longer to achieve orgasm.

- The labia majora (outer lips of the vagina) become thinner, paler, and slightly smaller.

- The breasts lose some of their firmness, fullness, and shape, and may even become slightly less sensitive.

- Clitoral stimulation may feel irritating, owing to lack of lubrication.

- The tissue of the urethra (the tube that carries urine from the bladder to outside the body), like the vagina, is estrogen dependent. As a result of declining estrogen levels, the urethra becomes thinner and more fragile. And because of its proximity next to the vagina, it is more likely to be traumatized during intercourse. All of these changes cause the urethra to become more vulnerable to bacteria, resulting in bladder infections.

- Pubic hair becomes less abundant.

While you may not experience all of them, these physical changes can affect your attitude toward sex because most of them lead to dyspareunia (painful sex). In addition to irritation, you may have itching, burning, pressure, and postcoital bleeding (vaginal bleeding after intercourse). And these problems, if not treated, can lead to other problems, including loss of sexual desire. After all, who wants to have sex if it hurts? Yet you want to maintain intimacy and closeness with your husband or partner.

Hormone replacement therapy (HRT) is the single most effective method of making intercourse pleasurable again. If you are unable to take HRT, you should not feel embarrassed if you take longer to lubricate; keep in mind that it also takes longer for a mature man to achieve erection.

Here are some steps you can take to help reduce discomfort and increase your enjoyment of sex:

- **Use a lubricant.** If vaginal dryness is your main problem, use a lubricant to prevent discomfort. Apply a generous amount to the vaginal opening just prior to intercourse. Never use a lubricant that is not designed for this specific purpose, especially oil-based products, such as petroleum jelly, cocoa butter, or baby oil. They tend to cake and dry and block the natural secretions you still produce. They can also create small holes in latex condoms (only latex condoms should be used for protection against sexually transmitted diseases [STDs]), and the holes allow viruses, bacteria, and sperm to pass through. Use only water-based lubricants made specifically for this purpose.

If you feel discomfort not only during penetration but also during active intercourse, try a lubricating vaginal suppository in addition to the lubricant gel. Start with the half-size suppositories, which may be enough, then move up to the full size if you find you need them.

- **Use a vaginal moisturizer.** There are nonhormonal vaginal moisturizers available that help the cells of the vaginal lining build up a moist protective layer. An added advantage is that these moisturizers have a very low pH. This means they are acidic and can therefore help maintain a healthy vaginal environment that discourages infection.

HRT still does a far superior job of restoring your vagina because it actually regenerates the protective layer of cells, thereby treating the underlying cause of the problem. But vaginal moisturizers significantly increase moisture and elasticity in the majority of women who use them. They are a useful alternative for treating vaginal dryness in those women past menopause who cannot or do not wish to take HRT.

• **Stay sexually active.** Regular sexual intercourse can help maintain your sexual responsiveness and keep your vagina more supple, elastic, and lubricated, lessening the likelihood that sex will become painful. Regular sexual activity (including masturbation, oral sex, manual stimulation, and the use of mechanical aids) increases the blood flow to your sexual organs, stimulates the glands that secrete lubrication, and slows the degenerative changes.

Many sexual problems are not hormonal, however, but are caused by such factors as poor communication between partners concerning their needs and desires, poor personal hygiene, unenthusiastic foreplay, or too little romance. Sex counseling or therapy (perhaps in addition to hormones) may be helpful in such cases.

• **Take a sitz bath.** Sitz baths will help to relieve acute irritation, itching, or burning. However, too much soaking will cause skin irritation.

• **Keep up those Kegel exercises.** To strengthen your pelvic floor muscles and improve vaginal tone, perform Kegel exercises as many times a day as you think of it (see page 29). Repeatedly squeeze and relax the muscles you would contract to stop urination. Or whenever you urinate, intermittently start and stop the flow, holding it for 10 seconds each time.

• **Take oral contraceptives.** If you are still having menstrual periods, even irregular ones, you still need protection against pregnancy. The low-dose combination birth control pill can serve as protection and, because it contains estrogen, can also help keep your vagina in good condition. Oral contraceptives will also keep irregular periods under control, making them predictable, and will suppress early perimenopausal symptoms.

• **Use vaginal estrogen cream.** If the moisturizers do not restore your vaginal lining enough to make sexual intercourse comfortable and you are not a candidate for HRT, then ask your doctor for a prescription for vaginal estrogen cream. Although this cream contains estrogen, very little of the hormone is absorbed into the bloodstream. How much and how often you use the cream depends on your needs. Some women do not absorb it as well as others and require a higher dose. Except in unusual cases, it is best to begin with one applicator at night for two to three nights per week until you see improvement, and then cut back to once a week as needed. You can maintain your own schedule with vaginal cream, starting and stopping it as necessary, but unless you start using another form of HRT, you will have to use the cream regularly to maintain a beneficial effect. Sometimes, even with HRT by tablet or patch, you will also need to use vaginal cream.

If you use estrogen cream, remember that some of the hormone is absorbed, so if you still have your uterus, your doctor may recommend that you also take progestin. If you decide not to take the progestin, you will need to visit your doctor regularly to be sure you are not developing endometrial hyperplasia (excessive thickening of the uterine lining), which can progress to cancer. If you are found to have hyperplasia, you must take progestin. Most importantly, report any bleeding that occurs while you are using an estrogen cream. Bleeding may indicate hyperplasia or other abnormal tissue inside the uterus.

Another device, now available, is an estrogen-releasing vaginal ring. The ring is placed in the vagina, much like a diaphragm, where it slowly releases minute amounts of estrogen that restore the vaginal lining and its ability to lubricate itself. The vaginal ring is designed to be replaced in the doctor's office or at home every 3 months.

• **Consider hormone replacement therapy.** Although all the above can go a long way toward relieving vaginal dryness and the subsequent decreased interest in sexual activity, estrogen replacement by pill or patch is the most effective treatment for these problems. Lubricants, moisturizers, and other measures do not supply estrogen, the key ingredient that restores the vagina's lining, its sensitivity, and its ability to provide lubrication when sexually stimulated. If you are having serious problems with your sex life and there is no medical reason you cannot take estrogen, talk to your doctor about HRT.

After starting HRT, you will see results in a couple of weeks when blood flow to the pelvic area increases, the vaginal lining begins to toughen and thicken, lubrication improves, and itchiness and soreness are relieved. And in a month or two, you will probably be back to normal. If, after taking HRT, you still have uncomfortable vaginal symptoms, see your doctor.

CHANGES IN DESIRE

Declining estrogen levels in midlife do not seem to affect sexual desire for most women, as long as intercourse remains comfortable and there are no other health-related problems to interfere with a healthy sex life.

However, some women lose interest in sex after menopause. This may be because of physical changes or because they never cared much for sex anyway or consider it an activity for younger people. Maybe more importantly, they may not have a partner who arouses them. After all, the best stimulus to sexual interest is a good lover. Many women have had unsatisfactory sexual relationships their entire lives and see menopause as a time when they are no longer expected to be sexually active. Also, some women's partners may have a chronic illness that affects sexual ability or desire. Other women, because of religious or social influences, believe that sexual activity is inappropriate except for the purpose of reproduction. Many women also repress their own sexual desires, responding only to their partner's sexual needs.

But many women, on the other hand, find that their interest in sex grows at midlife. Their early inhibitions seem to fade along with the demands of children, the burden of contraception, and the fear of pregnancy.

There are physical reasons why women may lose the desire for sexual relations. They include declining testosterone (the male sex hormone) levels and aging-related health problems.

The Role of Testosterone

One hormone thought to be responsible, at least in part, for sexual arousal is testosterone. It influences the libido in both men and women. Men produce about 10 times as much testosterone as women, but the hormone is thought to play an important role in the female sex drive. Although testosterone is present in females prior to menopause, its effects are tempered by the larger proportions of estrogen and progesterone.

However, the total amount of testosterone decreases at menopause, and, as a result, a woman may experience a dramatic loss of interest in sex and difficulty achieving orgasm.

Discuss with your doctor whether you can take a small amount of testosterone orally, either alone or in conjunction with your HRT regimen. A tiny dose of testosterone taken with HRT may help rekindle sexual feelings and improve your ability to reach orgasm. A blood test to check your testosterone level before or after treatment is not necessary.

The most common side effects of testosterone, noticed by a small percentage of women, are slight growth of hair on the chin and upper lip and an increased oiliness of the skin. Since many menopausal women report dry skin, the latter is not usually a problem. Facial hair is easily removable by plucking and does not persist if the testosterone therapy is stopped. For more information about testosterone, see Chapter 5.

Remember that many sexual problems are not caused by hormonal changes and that menopause need not result in loss of sexual desire. Besides the reasons listed above, lack of sexual interest may also result from poor communication between sex partners concerning their needs and desires, poor personal hygiene, or too little romance. Today there are a number of self-help methods available to help individuals and couples overcome problems with sexual desire. Videos and books can be found in stores and libraries or ordered through catalogs. If self-help is not for you, perhaps a professional counselor or therapist can help. Ask your doctor to recommend someone.

AGING-RELATED PROBLEMS

Factors associated with aging may often contribute to a decrease in sexual desire. Chronic health problems—such as cancer, arthritis, and heart disease—in a woman or her partner can affect sexual activity and desire.

Below is a description of some aging-related problems that can interfere with sexual activity.

Heart disease. Heart disease does not directly affect either partner's sexual responsiveness or ability to achieve orgasm. However, men and women with heart problems often fear that strenuous sexual activity may trigger a heart attack or a bout of angina (pain in the chest, arm, or jaw caused by lack of oxygen to the heart muscle). While orgasm does increase heart rate and blood pressure, it rarely leads to a heart attack. If this fear continues to get in the way of your enjoyment of sex, you may want to discuss the problem with your doctor.

Arthritis. The joint pain and reduced range of motion of arthritis can interfere with the physical mechanics of sexual intercourse. If this is the case, you may need to experiment with new positions in which to have intercourse. Sometimes firmer support, such as a board under the mattress or prop-up pillows or cushions under the pelvis, can help.

Osteoporosis. If you have osteoporosis, you can still have sex. You should, however, make sure that you have adequate vaginal lubrication. If you have vaginal dryness, try a lubricant, moisturizer, or HRT. If you have osteoporosis, HRT may be the best solution for you. It will relieve vaginal dryness and help prevent further bone loss.

Medications. Antihistamines and certain decongestants, designed to dry the mucous membranes of your nasal passages, will also dry out your vagina, so use them sparingly. Other drugs, including cardiovascular medications, antidepressants, atropine drugs, and diuretics may have the same effect. If you are taking any of these types of medication and your vagina seems dry, talk to your doctor about the possibility of changing or adjusting your medication.

Cancer. The psychological and physical effects of cancer can have a serious effect on a person's ability or desire to have sex. Drug regimens, as well as radiation therapy, have several side effects that can make a person feel sick most of the time.

In addition, cancer surgery (such as mastectomy or hysterectomy) can affect a woman's self-image, leading to decreased sexual desire. Surgical procedures such as breast reconstruction after mastectomy, as well as counseling and encouragement, can significantly reduce the impact. And so can education of both a woman and her partner. Both parties may be reassured after discussing with their doctor when it is safe to begin having sexual intercourse again.

Lack of a partner. One of the most overlooked sexual problems of older women is lack of a partner. A woman who reaches age 65 can expect to live for another 19 years; a man at 65 is expected to live only 14 more years. In addition, most women marry older men, thereby increasing the chances that a woman's husband will die before she does, leaving her alone for a number of years of widowhood. And the older a woman gets, the harder it can be for her to get out and meet people. Loss of mobility, health problems, fear of crime, and other isolating factors may cause her to avoid leaving her home unless it is absolutely necessary.

9

Gynecologic Problems and Procedures

This chapter describes some of the gynecologic problems and procedures that women may encounter in the years just before and after menopause. They include abnormal bleeding, pelvic support problems, stress incontinence and bladder instability, uterine cancer, ovarian cancer, and hysterectomy.

ABNORMAL BLEEDING

Once you reach menopause, menstrual periods have stopped. Once you have gone a year without periods, your menopause is complete. You will never have periods again, unless you are on hormone replacement therapy (HRT) that includes progestin.

If you are on this type of HRT, you should have light regular periods (called "withdrawal bleeding") just after you stop taking

AN ANATOMY OVERVIEW

To understand some of the gynecologic problems that can occur and the procedures you may need, it is helpful to be familiar with female anatomy.

The two ovaries are located on either side of the uterus, just above your pubic bone. The uterus lies in the pelvis, behind the urinary bladder. The uterus is a hollow organ about the size and shape of a small upside-down pear. It is made up of an outer muscular layer called the myometrium and an inner glandular lining, the endometrium. The main body of the uterus is the corpus. The cervix forms a canal that connects the cavity of the uterus with the top of the vagina.

Urine trickles slowly from the two kidneys down a pair of thin tubes called the ureters into the bladder, where it is stored. When urine is eliminated, it leaves the bladder through a short opening called the urethra. The floor of the pelvis is composed of strong connective tissue and the pelvic-floor muscles. These muscles support and surround the bladder, the urethra, the vagina, and the rectum.

the progestin each month. The purpose of the progestin is to balance the effect of the estrogen on the lining of the uterus by limiting its growth. These periods should be short (2 to 5 days) and have light to normal flow; however, the first few months that you take HRT, you might experience heavy flow while your body adjusts to the medications.

If any bleeding occurs at any time other than those few days, consider it abnormal and see your doctor right away. If the bleeding lasts longer than normal, if it does not occur on schedule, or if it is very heavy, report it to your doctor at once.

If you are not on HRT and you ever experience vaginal bleeding after menopause, call your doctor right away.

During perimenopause (the transition time before menopause that usually lasts 3 to 6 years), irregular uterine bleeding can be common. This bleeding is caused by the hormonal changes taking

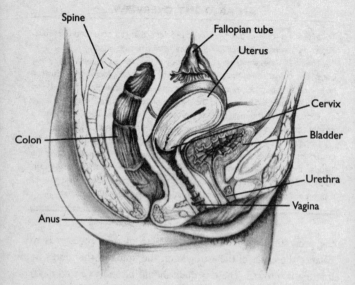

Female internal anatomy

place in your body, as your ovaries age and are less able to produce regular cyclic levels of estrogen and progesterone.

These changing hormone levels are due to failure to ovulate regularly and efficiently with each cycle, and, as a result, your menstrual bleeding patterns may change. You can expect an occasional period that is longer and heavier in flow. However, if this occurs more than once or twice and the flow is excessive, consult your doctor.

In general, if your periods come closer together than every 21 days (counting from the first day of one menstrual period to the first day of the next), if they last more than 7 days, if you bleed between periods, or if your periods become much heavier than they used to be, consult your doctor. Also, see your doctor if you have not had a period for 2 months.

If you see your doctor about abnormal bleeding, he or she will want to determine the cause. The visit may begin with a discussion to compare your present menstrual pattern with your previous menstrual pattern. So, before your appointment, try to recall the dates for and characteristics of your menstrual pattern over at least the last 2 or 3 months. It is always a good idea to keep a diary or journal of your menstrual cycles, especially at this stage of your life. By doing so, you alert yourself to abnormal changes as soon as they occur. And it helps you to better communicate problems to your doctor.

When treating a woman with abnormal vaginal bleeding, most doctors feel that the safest approach is to rule out any underlying disease—especially cancer. Procedures your doctor may perform to rule out problems include a Pap smear, ultrasound, endometrial biopsy, hysteroscopy, and sometimes, dilation and curettage (D & C) (see Common Gynecologic Procedures, pages 198 through 200).

Common causes of abnormal bleeding include hormonal fluctuations and imbalances, uterine fibroids, and endometrial polyps. Hyperplasia and endometrial cancer are less common causes of abnormal bleeding but are much more serious. The first three are discussed below. Hyperplasia and endometrial cancer are discussed on pages 212 through 218.

HORMONAL FLUCTUATIONS

The most common cause of abnormal bleeding in perimeno-pausal women is hormonal fluctuations that result from an imbalance of estrogen and progesterone. When you have cycles in which ovulation does not occur (meaning no egg is released), you do not produce any progesterone. The unopposed estrogen (unopposed in the sense that its effects are not counterbalanced by progesterone) causes a buildup of the lining of the uterus, which then sheds irregularly. It is the estrogen without sufficient progesterone that causes the heavy bleeding in this situation. This problem can sometimes be diagnosed by vaginal ultrasound (in which you hold a wand in your vagina while the technician takes the pictures) but is more commonly diagnosed by endometrial biopsy, which is discussed on page 199. This is because only a sample of actual tissue from inside the uterus can reliably confirm that there is no precancerous or cancerous condition of the uterine lining.

UTERINE FIBROIDS

Many women over age 30 have fibroids of the uterus; 30 percent to 50 percent of women have them by the time they reach age 50. Fibroids are benign (noncancerous) growths composed of uterine tissue that can sometimes grow to be very large. They can grow in the cavity of the uterus (submucosal), within the uterine wall (intramural), or on its outer surface (extramural). Where they are found often determines the symptoms they cause to a greater degree than does their size. Some women have only one or two fibroids, but it is more common to have several. Fibroids are most commonly diagnosed between ages 35 and 45. After menopause, fibroids may shrink because of declining estrogen levels.

Fibroids can range in size from tiny to larger than a grapefruit. They are seldom very painful unless very large and are not inherently dangerous or precancerous. Symptoms of fibroids include pressure and sometimes mild pain in the lower back or abdomen and heavy or long periods. Sometimes submucosal fibroids will cause excessive bleeding with periods. Taking a low-dose birth control pill will sometimes help control the bleeding. This treatment is useful with small fibroids, particularly if it can save a woman from having a hysterectomy. Submucosal fibroids can be identified by vaginal ultrasound or hysteroscopy and small ones can sometimes be removed (myomectomy) or at least reduced in size at the time of hysteroscopy with an instrument called a resectoscope. This is an outpatient procedure usually performed in an operating room. Large or multiple fibroids usually require a more extensive surgical procedure.

Fibroids are often identified during a routine pelvic examination, when your doctor feels them in your abdomen or sees them through the examining instrument. A vaginal or abdominal ultrasound may be performed to confirm the diagnosis.

Fibroids generally grow slowly. More rapid growth of fibroids may occur during pregnancy, stimulated by higher levels of estrogen. However, the low doses of estrogen used in HRT usually do not affect fibroid growth.

Even if fibroids do not cause bleeding, they can cause other problems. Large fibroids can press on your bladder, so that it can hold only small amounts of urine and you feel as though you have to urinate more often. Large fibroids can also place pressure on

COMMON GYNECOLOGIC PROCEDURES

In an attempt to evaluate conditions of the uterus, doctors use a number of different diagnostic tests or procedures, such as Pap smear, hysteroscopy, endometrial biopsy, and, less often, dilation and curettage (D & C). These procedures are explained below.

Pelvic examination and Pap smear. At this point in your life, you have already had many pelvic examinations and Pap smears. A pelvic examination is often performed as part of a physical checkup.

For the examination, you lie on your back on an examining table, with your knees bent and your feet in stirrups. An instrument called a speculum is inserted into your vagina to hold it open while your doctor uses a light to look for any abnormalities of the cervix and vaginal walls. He or she then scrapes some cells from the opening of the cervix and sends them to a laboratory. There, they are examined for conditions that might lead to cancer and for signs of cancer of the cervix. This procedure is called a Pap smear (after the man who developed it, G. N. Papanicolaou).

After taking the cells, the doctor removes the speculum, inserts one or two gloved fingers of one hand into your vagina, and carefully feels for any abnormalities of the uterus, ovaries, and fallopian tubes. He or she may perform a rectal exam also, to check for abnormal growths and blood in the stool.

The results of a Pap smear usually are known in a few weeks. The results are negative if the cells are normal and positive if they are precancerous or cancerous. Occasionally, the results are abnormal but inconclusive, and your doctor will recommend that the test be repeated in 3 months or he or she may perform a colposcopy. This is an examination of the cervix performed with a magnifying lens and a very bright light to determine the possible source of the abnormal cells, which is then biopsied. If the results indicate cancerous or precancerous cells, your doctor will arrange for further tests and treatment.

You should have a Pap smear at least every year—more often if your doctor recommends it. More frequent Pap smears may be recommended if you have ever been treated for a precancerous condition of the cervix or if you have any other condition that puts you at higher risk of cervical cancer. Some doctors may recommend a Pap smear test every 6 months for women on HRT.

Hysteroscopy. A hysteroscope is a flexible, or rigid, lighted viewing instrument that is inserted through the vagina, through the cervical canal, and into the uterus. Hysteroscopy is the name of the procedure using this instrument; it can be performed in a doctor's office or an outpatient surgicenter of a hospital using a local anesthetic. More complicated types of hysteroscopy, such as for removal of abnormal tissue (for example, a fibroid), are usually performed in an operating room.

A hysteroscopy allows a doctor to view the uterus directly and to evaluate and diagnose certain uterine disorders. It may, for example, confirm the presence of submucosal uterine fibroids, endometrial polyps, hyperplasia (thickening of the lining of the uterus), and abnormal growths of tissue. A hysteroscope may be used as a viewing aide during a D & C (see below) and can also be used to look for lost intrauterine devices (IUDs).

Hysterosalpingography. The imaging technique of hysterosalpingography is used to check for changes in the size and shape of a woman's uterus and fallopian tubes. Dye is injected into the uterus to outline the cavity of the uterus and the fallopian tubes, and an X ray is taken.

Ultrasound. Ultrasound, a painless imaging technique, uses sound waves to create a picture of the pelvic organs on a video screen. In abdominal ultrasound, a device called a transducer is moved across the abdomen to produce images of organs such as the uterus and kidneys. In vaginal ultrasound, a thin wand is inserted into the vagina to produce images of the ovaries and other reproductive organs. Ultrasound is used to evaluate and diagnose conditions such as polyps and submucosal fibroids. Ultrasound may also be performed after saline solution is injected into the uterine cavity. This technique is called sonohysterography.

Endometrial biopsy. In endometrial biopsy, a small sample of tissue is taken from the uterine lining and sent to a laboratory for examination under a microscope. A narrow catheter about the size of the lead in a pencil is passed through the cervical canal into the uterus to retrieve the tissue. Performed in your doctor's office, the procedure takes only a couple of minutes and may be uncomfortable but tolerable. Cramping may occur during and after the procedure. Endometrial biopsy is the easiest way to evaluate abnormal bleeding for cancer and hormonal imbalance.

Dilation and curettage (D & C). Rarely used anymore in favor of simpler, newer techniques, a D & C is a surgical procedure that scrapes away the uterine lining to determine the cause of frequent or heavy periods, to terminate a pregnancy, or to treat an incomplete abortion or miscarriage.

The procedure is usually performed under local anesthesia with sedation. The cervical canal is gradually dilated, the lining of the uterus is removed with a curet (a spoon-shaped surgical instrument), and the tissue samples are sent to a laboratory to be examined under a microscope. The procedure takes about 15 to 30 minutes.

After the procedure, slight bleeding from the uterus is possible for the first few days, and you may experience some cramping. You are usually able to go home the same day.

Sexual intercourse and use of tampons should be avoided for several days after a D & C, but most other activities can be resumed the next day, as long as you feel up to it. Any other problems should be discussed with your doctor right away.

---

your rectum, so that you feel as though you need to have a bowel movement. They can cause pain or pressure during intercourse. In addition, they can cause bloating or abdominal swelling or block the openings of the fallopian tubes and cause infertility. But they are not cancerous and they do not spread; the main problem is discomfort.

Often, if you have no discomfort, treatment of fibroids is conservative, especially during perimenopause. If a fibroid is just beginning to cause abnormal menstrual function or other problems at age 50, for example, it may require only another year of watchful waiting—prior to menopause—to get by without treatment. After menopause, when estrogen levels decline, fibroids tend to get smaller or even disappear. If your doctor recommends hysterectomy for fibroids (or any reason other than cancer), seek a second opinion. Your choice depends on your age, your symptoms, and your general health.

POLYPS

Cervical and endometrial polyps are benign (noncancerous) growths in the canal of the cervix and on the lining of the uterus, respectively. Polyps usually are single, but they may be multiple and can grow up to almost 1 inch in width. They may cause no symptoms at all, if small, or they may cause abnormal bleeding between periods, after sexual intercourse, or after menopause. Cervical polyps are usually detected during a routine physical examination. Endometrial polyps can be diagnosed in the course of an evaluation for abnormal bleeding, either by endometrial biopsy or ultrasound.

If you have an endometrial polyp, it should be removed for close examination in case it is premalignant (precancerous) and to relieve bleeding. The procedure to remove a polyp is quick and painless. The doctor snips it out easily through a hysteroscope (a viewing instrument).

PELVIC SUPPORT PROBLEMS

Over the course of your life, various symptoms can occur as a result of weakness in the supporting ligaments near your vagina, vulva, bladder, rectum, and uterus. These structures have usually been damaged or weakened during a vaginal delivery, or as a result of multiple pregnancies. Occasionally, these problems are hereditary.

As you age, the ligaments supporting the pelvic organs and the muscles in the pelvic area can become weaker and eventually lead to pelvic defects that involve prolapses, or "dropping," of the various organs. The prolapses vary in degree depending on the amount of damage to the structures involved. Prolapses usually occur in combination, although they occasionally occur as single events. The three types of prolapses are called cystocele, the dropping of the bladder into the vagina; rectocele, a pushing inward of the rectum into the vagina; and uterine prolapse, a dropping of the entire uterus due to weakness of the supports of the uterus itself.

Cystocele

A defect in the bladder and urethral supports within the upper walls of the vagina results in a prolapse of these organs into the vagina. Symptoms may include a sensation of pressure against the bladder or stress incontinence (an uncontrollable loss of a small amount of urine when coughing, laughing, or sneezing). Recurrent urinary tract infections, such as cystitis (a bladder infection), are also commonly associated with a cystocele. With large cystoceles, urinary frequency occurs due to incomplete bladder emptying. Your doctor can diagnose these conditions by pelvic examination.

Surgery is usually the treatment of choice if you are experiencing severe stress incontinence, the cystocele is rapidly enlarging, or you have had recurrent bouts of cystitis. Surgery involves a vaginal operation in which the defects are corrected by strengthening the muscles and ligaments that support these organs.

Rectocele

Rectocele is a pushing inward of the rectum toward the vagina due to weakness of the supporting muscles and ligaments. The defect usually originates after a difficult vaginal delivery and develops slowly over years. A rectocele usually does not cause symptoms until it becomes large, and then it may be difficult to fully empty the rectum when you have a bowel movement.

Your doctor can diagnose a rectocele during a pelvic examination. Treatment is surgical; a vaginal reconstruction operation is necessary to repair the damaged tissues.

Uterine Prolapse

The uterus, vagina, and other organs are held in place by strong muscles and ligaments at the base of the pelvis. As you get older, especially if you have had a few children and/or difficult vaginal deliveries, the muscles and ligaments that support the uterus and other pelvic organs become extremely stretched, weakened, or torn, allowing the uterus to sag. The weakening of the muscles may also occur as a result of decreased estrogen, as occurs at menopause, which may weaken the supporting tissues. In some cases, the muscles and ligaments no longer hold the uterus in place, so it falls and causes the vagina to sag downward. This causes the prolapse, a bulging of the front or back wall of the vagina. Sometimes the uterus may fall so far that it bulges out of the vagina, a condition referred to as complete prolapse.

A mild prolapse produces no annoying symptoms, but as the uterus falls lower, it may cause a heavy sensation in the vagina. If it becomes severe, a uterus can drop so that it feels like something is falling out. Uterine prolapse may cause stress incontinence or it may make urination more difficult. In addition, bowel movements may be difficult.

Mild prolapse is common, especially in later life. It can be uncomfortable and inconvenient, but there are few risks to your general health.

You can prevent pelvic relaxation to some degree by doing Kegel exercises to strengthen the muscles of the pelvic floor. See page 29 for a full description of how to do them. It also helps to maintain your ideal body weight. Too much weight can increase the abdominal pressure on your uterus.

If you experience a uterine prolapse, there are a few things you can do to lessen the symptoms. Lose weight if you are overweight. Eat plenty of high-fiber foods so that you will be able to move your bowels without straining. Continue to practice Kegel exercises throughout your life.

If there is no improvement, your doctor may recommend HRT to help strengthen the pelvic-floor muscles. Or he or she may recommend that you use a pessary, a rubber, ringlike device. It fits around the cervix to help prop up the sagging uterus and keep it from protruding into the vagina. Combined with estrogen cream and exercises to strengthen the pelvic floor, a pessary is effective for many women; however, it is inconvenient. The device must be carefully fitted by a doctor and then removed periodically for cleaning. Some women find it interferes with sexual intercourse and causes vaginal irritation that can lead to infection and bleeding.

Another option for uterine prolapse is surgery, usually a hysterectomy, in which the uterus is removed through the vagina. In fact, about 15 percent of all hysterectomies are performed for this reason. An advantage to surgery is that at the same time, a prolapsed bladder or rectum can be repositioned and its vaginal supports tightened.

URINARY INCONTINENCE

The urinary tract is made up of the kidneys, ureters (two long tubes from the kidneys to the bladder), the bladder (which stores the urine produced in the kidneys), and the urethra (the passageway from the bladder to the outside of the body), which emerges very close to the opening of the vagina.

Urinary incontinence (leakage of urine) affects millions of Americans of all ages and both sexes. It is a problem that occurs naturally with aging and after childbirth. More common in women than in men, it is probably related to menopause.

Up to one fourth of all adult women are incontinent to some extent. Some researchers believe that almost half of women over age 45 have the problem at least occasionally. Women are more likely to have leaky bladders if they have had children, and the incidence rises rapidly with age.

It is not normal to be incontinent, no matter how old you are. Incontinence is not a disease but rather a symptom of an underlying condition that can often be corrected. Factors leading to incontinence may include recurrent infections, lack of estrogen after menopause, weak pelvic muscles, a sagging bladder, muscle damage during childbirth, or obesity. Treat the underlying condition, and the problem may be solved.

If you have urinary incontinence, the first thing you need to do is talk to your doctor. The treatment that is appropriate for you depends on the kind and degree of urinary incontinence you have, as well as the reason you have it. Almost all cases of incontinence among older women are either of the following types.

Stress incontinence. The most common form of urinary incontinence is stress incontinence. It is characterized by episodes in which an involuntary spurt of urine escapes the bladder when you laugh, sneeze, cough, lift an object, exercise, or stand up quickly. Usually caused by a weakened urethral sphincter (the ring of muscle that regulates outflow of urine) or a sagging urethra that allows urine to seep out when the abdomen exerts pressure on the bladder, stress incontinence tends to get worse after menopause when your estrogen level drops. This sagging or prolapse of the urethra and bladder is accompanied by prolapse of the rectum or uterus and happens most frequently in women who delivered their children vaginally.

Urge incontinence (bladder instability). Urge incontinence is the uncontrollable need to urinate accompanied by inability to control the bladder.

What Causes Urinary Incontinence?

Like many other parts of the body, the bladder and urethra change as you get older. The muscles of the bladder tend to weaken and the bladder wall becomes stiffer, decreasing its ability to expand.

At menopause, with the loss of estrogen, the bladder loses additional muscle tone and elasticity, making it less able to hold as much urine as it once did. The outermost portion of the urethra also becomes less flexible and elastic and therefore becomes more at risk for injury and infection. Blood flow to the area decreases. Also, the walls of the vagina shrink after menopause and provide less support for the urethra and bladder. Sometimes, in severe cases of estrogen deficiency, the urethra prolapses, sagging into the vagina. All of these factors combine to lower the ability of the bladder and urethra to hold back urine when you cough, laugh, or sneeze.

Other causes of urinary incontinence include the following.

Weakened pelvic muscles. The pelvic floor—the muscles that encircle and support the urethra, vagina, and rectum—often become stretched and less supportive because of pregnancies, childbirth, previous surgery, normal aging, and a lack of estrogen. Then, as a result, the bladder and urethra drop lower in the pelvis, where they become less able to hold urine under pressure.

Urinary tract infection. When the bladder is infected, it may become extremely irritated, which causes it to contract, making it less able to hold urine.

Obesity. Being overweight increases abdominal pressure on the bladder.

Medications and food. Medications, such as antihypertensives and antidepressants, and foods, such as sugar, coffee, alcohol, artificial sweeteners, and spicy dishes, sometimes cause incontinence as a side effect, especially when pelvic muscles are already weakened.

What to Do

Your doctor can make a diagnosis of incontinence with a complete physical and neurologic examination, a urinalysis to check for infection, bladder-function tests, and perhaps a cystoscopy (a close examination of the bladder and urethra with the help of a lighted instrument that is passed through the urethra). In addition, he or she may ask you to keep a diary for a few days, noting your trips to the bathroom, the amount of urine, episodes of incontinence, the food you eat, your daily routine, and the medications you take.

HRT will definitely help, but it may not cure your incontinence. Estrogen replacement can restore the bladder and urethral tissue to a state that is a lot closer to its former self. If you do not want to take oral estrogen in the form of HRT because of its risks, your doctor can prescribe vaginal estrogen cream. Applied to the skin of the vagina, the cream's effects are almost completely limited to the vagina and the urethra. You may still need to take progestin if you have your uterus, however, to help prevent endometrial cancer.

Sometimes simple changes in diet or the elimination of certain drugs can cure you or at least greatly improve the situation. Often, clearing up an infection with antibiotics will do it. Sometimes the problem is solved by behavioral techniques, such as bladder training, muscle-strengthening exercises, biofeedback, or frequent trips to the bathroom. Other treatments include medications to increase bladder capacity, relax the bladder, or stimulate contractions.

Usually, a combination of treatments and self-help measures is used. An important point to remember in the treatment of incontinence is that it takes time, but there may be a remarkable improvement if you just work at it. The usual treatments include the following:

• **Hormone replacement therapy.** Hormone replacement is usually used in combination with other treatments, although by itself, it may cure mild cases of stress incontinence. HRT is frequently prescribed before pelvic surgery to restore the tissues to their optimal condition before the operation.

• **Bladder training.** Bladder training teaches you to urinate only at scheduled times, with gradually increasing intervals between trips to the bathroom. For example, to train your bladder, you begin by going to the bathroom by the clock every 30 to 60 minutes during your waking hours, whether or not you feel the need, resisting urges to urinate at unscheduled times, and then urinating on schedule, whether you feel the need. After about a week, you increase the time between trips by half an hour, continuing to increase the interval by half-hourly increments every week or so until, after about 6 weeks, you have trained your bladder to wait at least 4 hours.

• **Kegel exercises.** As described in Chapter 3, Kegel exercises are designed to strengthen the muscles that support the base of the bladder. These exercises can often alleviate stress incontinence. You must first get the feel for tightening the proper muscles, the same muscles that are used to stop the flow of urine in midstream.

Whenever you think of it, as many times a day as possible, exercise these muscles. While doing so, keep the muscles relaxed in your abdomen, buttocks, and thighs.

As you get in the habit of doing these exercises, keep in mind that it usually takes a few months of faithful exercising to strengthen the muscles enough to tighten your urethra. And then you must keep it up. If you stop exercising, the muscles will relax again.

• **Double voiding.** Because it is important to empty your bladder completely when you urinate, which is difficult for many women, get in the habit of urinating, waiting a few minutes, then going again. Or stand up, bend over, walk around, rub your lower abdomen, and then sit down and finish urinating.

- **Medications.** Drugs can increase the bladder's ability to hold urine by decreasing its involuntary contractions or by tightening the sphincter muscle. Some drugs—for example, oxybutynin—are designed to block involuntary bladder contractions. Another decreases urine production. Others tighten the muscles around the urethra. Often, these medications work best when they are used in combination with HRT.

- **Biofeedback.** Biofeedback helps you learn to regulate your urinary tract. You need to see a specialist to receive biofeedback treatment. Consult your doctor.

- **Treatment of infection.** Other medications, such as antibiotics, can cure underlying infections that may be causing the incontinence.

- **Drug avoidance.** Some medications, including several used to control hypertension, have been linked to leakage problems. Ask your doctor about potential side effects whenever he or she gives you a prescription. Other medications that can cause problems for women are sedatives, diuretics, antidepressants, antihistamines, and decongestants.

- **Surgery.** If other treatments fail, surgery can be remarkably effective for stress incontinence. It can correct structural abnormalities, reposition a sagging bladder and urethra, strengthen the supporting ligaments, remove obstructions, bolster weakened muscles, and replace a defective sphincter.

As you work to find which of the above treatments can help relieve your incontinence, there are a number of things you can do yourself to help deal with the problem.

- **Drink a lot of liquids.** You might think it would be a good idea to cut back on your fluid intake in the hopes that you will not have to urinate so often. But the smaller amount of urine you produce when you are dehydrated may be more highly concentrated, which makes it irritating to the bladder and more likely to encourage bacterial infections. Do not cut back on liquids unless your doctor advises it. Dehydration can also cause many other health problems. However, do not drink a lot of fluids late in the evening. This may cause you to get up several times during the night to urinate.

- **Lose excess weight.** Taking off a few pounds can make a big difference, as it takes excess pressure off your bladder and urethra.

- **Stop smoking.** Women who smoke have more than double the risk of urinary incontinence than nonsmokers. Not only does smoking irritate the bladder lining and damage nerves, but it is also associated with bladder cancer. It also makes you cough, which could lead to leakage of urine.

- **Watch the foods you eat.** Try eliminating foods that are bladder irritants, such as alcohol, carbonated beverages, caffeine, milk, citrus fruits, tomatoes, spicy foods, sugar, honey, chocolate, and artificial sweeteners.

- **Watch what you use.** Avoid colored or perfumed toilet paper and feminine hygiene products, detergent bath additives, and perfumed soaps. All of these products help promote allergic reactions or sometimes infection.

- **Eat a high-fiber diet.** Fiber helps to prevent constipation. Consuming a lot of fruits and vegetables may also help prevent bladder cancer.

- **Never strain during a bowel movement.** If you have trouble with constipation, increase your fiber intake. Stool softeners, which help increase the water content in the stool, are available over the counter and are safe to use. Ask your doctor for advice on dealing with constipation.

• **Avoid heavy lifting.** Lifting heavy objects strains the pelvic floor muscles and puts pressure on the bladder and urethra.

HYPERPLASIA AND ENDOMETRIAL CANCER

Endometrial cancer is highly curable if it is caught early—before it has a chance to spread beyond the uterus. It is critical to understand that successful treatment is possible only with early diagnosis. This means that all women, especially those in menopause, must watch for any symptoms. This provides the best chances of early detection and successful treatment.

Cancer of the endometrium appears most often around or after menopause. The most common symptom is usually abnormal vaginal bleeding. After menopause—when normal menstrual bleeding has stopped—any bleeding, unless you are on cyclic HRT, is considered abnormal. The bleeding may be very light and sporadic or it may be heavy. If you experience any bleeding that you are not expecting, see your doctor right away. If the disease progresses unnoticed to a more advanced stage, symptoms can include pelvic pain or abdominal swelling. Luckily, it is usually discovered before it reaches this point.

What Is Endometrial Cancer?

Cancer is abnormal tissue growth brought about by an uncontrolled division of cells. In endometrial cancer, the tissue involved is the lining of the cavity of the uterus.

Without order, these cells multiply, pile up, and eventually form excess tissue that has no function except to grow. As the tissue increases, it forms tissue masses known as tumors. Some are benign (not likely to spread) and some are malignant (likely to spread). Cancerous tumors can destroy normal uterine tissue and break away to spread from one organ to another, invading other parts of the body. This spreading is called metastasis.

Who Is at Risk?

As with most cancers, how and why endometrial cancer develops remains a mystery. Your chances of developing endometrial cancer are greater if you:

- Began menstruating at an early age
- Went through menopause late (after age 52)
- Are considerably overweight
- Have never had a full-term pregnancy
- Have chronic lack of ovulation prior to menopause

While endometrial cancer does not appear to be inherited, there is a tendency for it to appear more often among relatives. Women who develop certain ovarian tumors, which secrete estrogen, are also at higher risk, as are women with endometrial hyperplasia (discussed below).

Diabetes and/or high blood pressure are also common in women who develop endometrial cancer, but the excess weight that accompanies these conditions is probably the cause of the problem. Women who are 50 pounds overweight are nine times as likely as women of normal weight to develop the disease. As you may recall, excess fatty tissue turns certain hormones into a form of estrogen, and women with high levels of estrogen are twice as likely to develop endometrial cancer.

Estrogen therapy or HRT is a factor in the development of endometrial cancer only if the estrogen is not combined with progestin. Estrogen alone can stimulate the endometrium to grow excessively and can increase the likelihood of endometrial hyperplasia, which in turn can progress to cancer. To reduce this risk, women are advised to take progestin with estrogen, which has been shown to reverse endometrial hyperplasia. Progestin therapy in conjunction with estrogen reduces the risk of endometrial cancer to less than the risk of a woman who takes no hormones.

A history of certain other diseases, such as polycystic ovarian disease, ovarian tumor, and colon or rectal cancer, also increases some women's chances of developing endometrial cancer. Women who have had breast cancer are more prone to develop endometrial cancer; and the breast-cancer drug tamoxifen has also been linked to an increased risk of endometrial cancer. In fact, any history of cancer of a woman's reproductive organs increases the risk of endometrial cancer.

Endometrial cancer is diagnosed in nearly 40,000 women each year in the US. It represents 6 percent of all cancers in women. It occurs more often than any other cancer of the reproductive tract, now exceeding cervical cancer.

As the US population ages, the number of endometrial cancer cases is increasing. However, the mortality rate from endometrial cancer is low: about 3 women in 100,000. The lower mortality rate for endometrial cancer—despite its higher incidence—is primarily a result of early detection. Because bleeding often provides clear warning early in the disease, the cancer can be caught while it is still confined to the uterus.

Endometrial Cancer's Early Beginnings: Hyperplasia

Hyperplasia is an excessive growth of endometrial cells. In hyperplasia, the uterine lining becomes thicker than it should. Catching hyperplasia early is important, as endometrial cancer almost always goes through a hyperplasia stage first.

Hyperplasia is not cancer, but it can be a precancerous condition. Among the few women predisposed to endometrial cancer, hyperplasia can develop into a malignancy (a tumor likely to spread) if left untreated. On the other hand, hyperplasia does not always turn into cancer, even if left untreated.

Hyperplasia usually causes bleeding at unscheduled times, or if you are not menopausal, it produces very heavy menstrual periods. If you see your doctor whenever you have irregular, unexpected, or extraheavy bleeding, you will be tested for hyperplasia with an endometrial biopsy, vaginal ultrasound, or, in some cases, D & C (see pages 199 through 200).

If your doctor determines that you have endometrial hyperplasia, you will first be treated with progestin. You will take progestin every day for 2 or 3 months, and then the endometrial biopsy is repeated to ensure that the treatment has been effective. If you still have hyperplasia, further investigation will be necessary.

Diagnosing Endometrial Cancer

You cannot be reminded enough: the single most important early warning sign associated with endometrial cancer is abnormal vaginal bleeding. However, not all abnormal bleeding is caused by endometrial cancer. Other possible causes of bleeding include hormonal fluctuations, noncancerous endometrial or cervical polyps, fibroids, and endometrial hyperplasia. Abnormal bleeding may also occur in women who have cervical cancer, ovarian cancer, or a rare type of uterine cancer known as uterine sarcoma.

If you are past menopause and experience any kind of bleeding from the vagina, you should have diagnostic tests to rule out endometrial and other types of cancer. If your doctor discovers endometrial cells on a Pap smear, you should also be evaluated for cancer. Even pre- and perimenopausal women who experience bleeding between periods or increasingly heavy, prolonged bleeding should be screened for this cancer, particularly if they have a history of anovulation (failure to ovulate). The tests and screenings performed to diagnose endometrial cancer are described on pages 217 through 218.

Classifying Endometrial Cancer

Like most cancers, endometrial cancer is classified by its stage. It can progress through five stages, from tissue abnormalities such as hyperplasia to cancer that has spread to the bladder, intestines, or other parts of the body, such as the cervix and vagina, the nearby lymph nodes, the abdominal cavity, and even more distant organs and lymph nodes. Cancer spreads to distant areas of the body by way of the lymphatic system. Therefore, it is vital that your doctor carefully checks the lymph nodes near the uterus and cervix, because apparently unaffected lymph nodes can still contain the cancer.

The stages of endometrial cancer include the following:

- **Stage 0:** The cancer is confined to the uterine lining and has not spread. Some doctors use this stage to refer to the most severe form of abnormal hyperplasia, called carcinoma in situ.

- **Stage I:** The cancer is confined to the uterus. Stage I cancers are further subdivided by the depth of invasion of the cancer into the uterine wall.
- **Stage II:** The cancer has spread to the cervix but not beyond the uterus.
- **Stage III:** The cancer has spread to the vagina and/or surrounding lymph nodes.
- **Stage IV:** The cancer has spread to the bladder and/or large intestine (colon) or to other organs beyond the pelvis.

Treating Endometrial Cancer

Treatment of endometrial cancer depends on whether you have hyperplasia or cancer and on the stage of the cancer. If an endometrial biopsy or hysteroscopy shows that you have hyperplasia, your doctor will recommend that you take progestin therapy. After progestin treatment, he or she will perform another endometrial biopsy to ensure that the treatment has been successful.

If hyperplasia persists after progestin therapy or if you have hyperplasia with abnormal cells, a hysterectomy (surgical removal of the uterus) is usually recommended.

For endometrial cancer, an abdominal hysterectomy and bilateral salpingo-oophorectomy (removal of the uterus, fallopian tubes, and ovaries) is the treatment of choice. The doctor will also take tissue samples from the lymph nodes in the pelvis and adjacent to the major blood vessels in the pelvis and abdomen to determine if the cancer has spread. Most doctors recommend that your ovaries be removed because women with endometrial cancer are at increased risk of developing ovarian cancer, which is much more difficult to detect in its early stages. See pages 222 through 226 for a description of these surgeries.

If cancer has spread to the lymph nodes or adjacent organs, you may need follow-up radiation therapy to prevent recurrence of the cancer in the vagina and lymph nodes.

Overall, the outlook for women with endometrial cancer is good. Most women with endometrial cancer are diagnosed in the early stages (stage I), when the survival rate is highest.

OVARIAN CANCER

Ovarian cancer accounts for a very small percentage of all cancers among women, but it is a leading cause of cancer death among women. This is largely because ovarian cancer is a "silent" disease, often causing no symptoms until the cancer is in an advanced stage. In fact, less than 30 percent of ovarian cancers are confined to the ovaries at the time they are diagnosed. Yet the cure rate for ovarian cancer that has not spread can be as high as 90 percent. Improved screening tests hold promise of detecting this cancer earlier and improving a woman's chances of surviving the disease.

Ovarian cancer is uncommon. Your overall chances of developing it are 1 in 80—in contrast to a breast cancer rate of 1 in 9. Even if you are in your fifties or sixties, which is the age group at greatest risk, your chances of developing ovarian cancer are still only 1 in 70.

The Symptoms

One reason ovarian cancer is so deadly is that it rarely shows any symptoms in its earlier stages. To compound the problem, because the ovaries are located deep within the abdomen, there is no way to do a self-examination. And when the disease does produce symptoms, they can often be confusing, possibly signaling many other conditions. However, if you have any unexplainable symptoms, see your doctor as soon as possible.

The most common symptoms of ovarian cancer are vague stomach discomfort, a swollen abdomen, or abnormal bleeding. Many women have these symptoms but do not report them to their doctor until the doctor feels an enlarged ovary during the course of a routine pelvic examination or the disease is in an advanced stage.

However, even when your doctor finds an ovarian growth, it does not always mean that you have cancer. In fact, the great majority of ovarian growths detected in premenopausal women are benign (not likely to spread) and eventually disappear on their own. If you are over age 50, an enlarged ovary is considered potentially more serious, because the ovary normally shrinks during menopause. Also, ovarian cancer occurs more frequently in women in their fifties and sixties. However, growths found in postmenopausal women are often benign (noncancerous) cysts.

Who's at Risk?

As with endometrial cancer and other cancers, no one knows for sure what causes the growth of cancerous ovarian cells. It is possible that a number of factors may influence their development, including the following:

- Age—women between ages 50 and 60 are at highest risk
- Never having been pregnant or having your first pregnancy after age 30
- Late menopause
- Family history of cancer

An important indicator of whether you are at risk of developing ovarian cancer is your family medical history. If your mother or sister has had ovarian cancer, your risk increases tenfold. A family history of endometrial or breast cancer appears to double your risk of ovarian cancer. A history of colon cancer, lung cancer, or prostate cancer in an immediate family member also increases your risk.

Oral contraceptives protect women against ovarian cancer. Women who take birth control pills for 10 years have an 80 percent reduction in the risk of ovarian cancer. Premenopausal women with a family history of the disease are often advised to consider taking oral contraceptives for this reason. Protection appears to begin in as little as 3 to 6 months of oral contraceptive use and continues for up to 15 years after you stop taking the pill.

Diagnosing Ovarian Cancer

If during an internal exam your doctor feels a growth that might indicate an enlarged ovary, he or she will usually recommend an ultrasound of the pelvic area. This painless diagnostic test allows your doctor to see your internal reproductive organs. Generally, if a growth is small and only one ovary is involved, the chances are very good that it is benign (noncancerous). However, you should still follow through with any further evaluation, testing, or treatment that your doctor recommends.

Certain blood tests are also helpful in making a diagnosis of cancer. For example, the type of ovarian cancers called epithelial (a certain type of cell) have been found to produce a protein known as CA-125. Therefore, a blood test that detects CA-125 can provide useful diagnostic information, especially in post-menopausal women. A higher level of this substance in the blood than normal, along with an ultrasound that shows an ovarian growth, can lead your doctor to recommend further testing. However, like many tests, the one for CA-125 levels can produce a false-positive result, predicting that a possible cancer is present when in fact the mass is benign. This is because other conditions, such as fibroid tumors or endometriosis (abnormal growth of endometrial tissue outside the uterus), can also cause elevated levels of CA-125, especially in premenopausal women.

If your doctor is still not sure about the nature of a pelvic growth, he or she will recommend that you undergo a laparoscopy (surgery performed through one to four small incisions [cuts] in the abdomen), in which a biopsy of the ovaries can be obtained. This is the only definitive way to make a diagnosis of ovarian cancer.

Treating Ovarian Cancer

If cancer of the ovaries is found, treatment involves surgical removal of both ovaries as well as of the uterus and fallopian tubes. Radiation and/or chemotherapy is recommended for women with cancer cells elsewhere in the pelvic cavity. Sometimes a second laparoscopy is performed several months later to see whether any cancer cells have been missed or have recurred. Periodic blood tests may be performed to monitor the side effects of the chemotherapy treatment.

GYNECOLOGIC SURGICAL PROCEDURES

Hysterectomy is the most frequently performed major surgical procedure in the US, aside from cesarian sections. The most common age at which this procedure is performed is 40 to 45.

While a hysterectomy can save your life if you have cancer of the reproductive organs, it is more often performed to treat such benign (noncancerous) conditions as fibroid tumors of the uterus, heavy periods, uterine prolapse, and endometriosis—conditions for which there are sometimes alternative forms of treatment.

There are many reasons why hysterectomies have declined in number since the late 1980s. Advances in conservative surgical procedures and hormonal treatment have given women other options. There are various types of gynecologic surgical procedures, classified according to which organs are removed during the operation.

Types of Procedures

Total abdominal hysterectomy. The uterus and cervix are removed through an incision (cut) in the abdomen. The ovaries are left in place. If you have a hysterectomy before menopause, you will still experience symptoms of menopause at the normal time, with one exception: you will not have the cessation of menstruation to indicate the arrival of menopause.

Subtotal, or supracervical, hysterectomy. The uterus above the cervix is removed. The cervix, ovaries, and fallopian tubes are left intact.

Oophorectomy. One ovary is removed. If you are not yet in menopause when you lose one ovary, the other ovary will take over, ovulating every month and producing the same levels of estrogen and progesterone necessary to regulate your menstrual cycle. You will be able to have children and you will experience natural menopause at the time you normally would have without the operation.

Salpingo-oophorectomy. One fallopian tube and ovary on one side is removed. Again, if the surgery is performed before menopause, the other ovary will compensate for the loss.

Bilateral oophorectomy. Both ovaries are removed. When performed before menopause, bilateral oophorectomy results in instantaneous, or surgical, menopause, regardless of whether the uterus is left intact.

Bilateral salpingo-oophorectomy. Both ovaries and fallopian tubes are removed. Bilateral salpingo-oophorectomy results in surgical menopause for premenopausal women.

Total abdominal hysterectomy with bilateral salpingo-oophorectomy. The uterus (with the cervix), both fallopian tubes, and both ovaries are removed. A total abdominal hysterectomy with bilateral salpingo-oophorectomy results in surgical menopause for premenopausal women.

Radical hysterectomy. Usually performed to treat invasive cancer of the cervix or endometrium, a radical hysterectomy involves the removal of the top third of the vaginal canal, the supporting tissues around the uterus, and the lymph glands that drain the pelvic area.

There are three ways in which a hysterectomy can be performed:

- **Abdominal hysterectomy.** The most common method, abdominal hysterectomy, involves the removal of the uterus through an incision made in the abdominal wall. This route must be taken when there are large fibroids or endometriosis; when cancer is suspected; when an examination of the ovaries or other internal organs is needed; when chronic infections may involve the fallopian tubes or ovaries; or when, because of previous surgery or infection, the uterus is surrounded by scar tissue.
- **Vaginal hysterectomy.** A vaginal hysterectomy involves removing the uterus through the vagina. It is usually reserved for uncomplicated conditions involving only the uterus, such as endometrial hyperplasia, abnormal uterine bleeding, and uterine prolapse. Because the uterus is removed through the vagina, there is no abdominal incision, no scar, less pain, and a slightly shorter hospitalization and recovery time.
- **Laparoscopically assisted vaginal hysterectomy.** In a laparoscopically assisted vaginal hysterectomy, the uterus is detached through one to four tiny abdominal incisions (cuts) with the help of a laparoscope (a small, lighted viewing instrument), then removed through the vagina. With the help of an external video monitor, the laparoscope provides the surgeon with a close-up view of the abdomen and uterus, giving him or her an opportunity to perform additional steps, such as removing any scar tissue in the abdomen. Postoperative pain and recovery time are similar to those of a vaginal hysterectomy.

Should Ovaries Be Removed Too?

If you are going to have a hysterectomy and are over age 40 to 45, your doctor may suggest that your ovaries be removed at the same time, even if they are healthy.

The argument for routinely removing ovaries in women who are approaching menopause is that they are not going to need their ovaries, because they will no longer be able to bear children, so it makes sense to eliminate the future risk of ovarian cancer.

The argument against removing healthy ovaries is that the risk of ovarian cancer is quite small—less than 2 percent. This risk must be measured against the major effects of losing all of your ovarian function. If you are still menstruating, having your ovaries removed produces instant menopause. You will probably have menopausal symptoms within a day or two of surgery, unless you begin HRT immediately after surgery.

The decision to remove or keep your healthy ovaries is yours to make. Be sure you know what your doctor plans to do, make sure you understand and agree with his or her opinion, and discuss your options. (Before consenting to surgery, read the questions below.)

QUESTIONS TO ASK BEFORE AGREEING TO HYSTERECTOMY

The decision to have any type of surgery is a serious one. Some surgeries have obvious benefits; others may not. If your doctor recommends that you have any organs of your reproductive system removed, you must ask yourself and your doctor some questions. You need to make an informed decision, by gathering as much information as you can. Ask your doctor why you need surgery, what will be removed, what are your alternatives, and what are the risks and benefits. Do not be afraid to ask these questions—it is your body and your decision to make.

Once you understand your doctor's recommendation, get a second opinion. Some programs requiring a second opinion before hysterectomy have reported a substantial decrease in the number of operations, suggesting that some hysterectomies may be unnecessary.

Before you consent to having surgery, be sure you are satisfied with your decision. If surgery is unavoidable (and in some cases it may be your only option), prepare yourself emotionally and physically.

Here are some good questions to ask before consenting to surgery. Modify them to suit your needs.

- Why do I need to have a hysterectomy?
- What organ or organs will be removed and why?
- Will my ovaries be left in place? If not, why not?
- Will my cervix be removed? If so, why?
- Are there alternatives for me besides a hysterectomy?
- What are the advantages, risks, and benefits of each alternative?
- What will be the physical effects of a hysterectomy?
- Are these effects permanent?
- What will happen to my weight, my breasts, and [anything else you want to ask about]?
- How will a hysterectomy affect my sex life?
- Will I experience menopause? Can the symptoms of menopause be treated? What are the risks and benefits of such treatment for me specifically?
- Will the operation be a vaginal, abdominal, or laparoscopically assisted hysterectomy?
- What can I expect in the hospital? What are the preoperative procedures? How long will I have to stay in the hospital? Related questions are about the type of anesthesia to be used, the risk of infection, the need for a blood transfusion, and donation of your own blood before surgery to be stored in the blood bank in case you need it later.
- What kind of care will I need after my hysterectomy?
- How should I prepare for coming home from the hospital?
- How soon will I be able to go back to work?
- When I can resume sexual activity?

Your Menopause Health Priorities Checklist

As you can see, there is a lot you can do to stay healthy before and after menopause. We hope that the information in this book encourages you to maintain a healthy lifestyle, educate yourself about menopause, work with your doctor, and make informed decisions about your health and health care. The following checklist provides brief descriptions of your health priorities and the most important things you can do to maintain your good health now and in the future.

- **Consider taking hormone replacement therapy.** Taking estrogen in the form of hormone replacement therapy (HRT) significantly decreases your risk of cardiovascular disease and stroke and also helps protect against osteoporosis, the debilitating bone disease (see Chapter 5). Talk to your doctor about taking HRT and be sure that you understand your options and the full range of benefits and risks before making your decision.

- **Keep your bones strong.** For strong, healthy bones (see pages 55 through 66), you need to consume between 1,000 and 1,500 milligrams of calcium every day. Also, regular weight-bearing exercises (for example, exercises such as jogging and step aerobics, which put stress on the large muscles of your lower body) can help you maintain the strength of your bones. Replacing estrogen in the form of HRT can significantly reduce your risk of osteoporosis.

• **Have regular mammograms.** As you age, your risk of breast cancer increases. Early detection and treatment are vital. Mammograms (see pages 69 and 94) can detect potentially cancerous breast lumps when they are too small to be felt by hand. You should have a baseline mammogram at age 40 and then have a regular mammogram every 1 to 2 years until age 50, when you should begin having a mammogram every year.

• **Follow a healthy diet.** A healthy diet (see page 132) provides essential nutrients, vitamins, minerals, and fiber and will help reduce your risk of cancer, osteoporosis, heart disease, and stroke. A healthy diet for women in menopause includes plenty of fruit, vegetables, whole grains, and low-fat, calcium-rich foods. Also, be sure to drink six to eight glasses of water, at least 8 ounces each, every day.

• **Exercise regularly.** Regular exercise (see pages 116 through 132) helps reduce your risk of aging-related diseases such as hypertension, heart disease, and stroke. Weight-bearing exercises (for example, exercises such as brisk walking and stair climbing, which put stress on the large muscles of your lower body) will help you maintain strong, healthy bones. Exercise can also help reduce stress and improve your overall sense of well-being. It's never too late to start exercising.

• **Take care of your heart.** Some of the steps you can take to lower your risk of heart disease (see page 50) are to stop smoking, eat a healthy diet, control high blood pressure, maintain a healthy weight, and control stress. Also, replacing estrogen in the form of HRT can reduce your risk of heart disease.

• **Have regular medical checkups.** It is especially important to maintain a good relationship with your doctor. See your doctor as often as he or she recommends for regular medical checkups that include a blood pressure check, a breast examination, a pelvic examination, and screening tests (for example, mammograms). Be sure to ask questions and get second opinions so that you can make informed decisions regarding your treatment options.

- **Avoid or manage stress.** Menopause is a stressful time of life, and stress can be a factor in diseases such as hypertension and depression. Some useful steps you can take to manage the stress (see pages 164 through 179) in your life include eating a healthy diet, exercising regularly, using relaxation techniques, and talking things over with your spouse or a close friend or relative. If you feel overwhelmed by the stress in your life, ask your doctor to refer you to a psychiatrist or other mental health professional.

- **Have a healthy sex life.** It is important for you to stay sexually active, if possible, and maintain intimacy with your spouse or partner (see Chapter 8). Be aware that physical changes in you or your spouse may affect your sexual relationship. Know what to expect from one another, keep the lines of communication open, and be patient. Many midlife sex problems can be effectively treated. Talk to your doctor if you have any concerns or questions.

Now that you have the reliable, up-to-date information that you need, the rest is up to you. We wish you many years of good health.

Glossary

This glossary defines terms that your doctor may have mentioned or that you may have come across while reading about menopause. Italicized words within entries refer you to other entries for additional information.

A

adrenal glands: Two triangular glands, one on top of each kidney, that produce a variety of hormones that affect nearly every body system.

aerobic exercise: Physical exercise that requires your heart and lungs to work harder to meet your muscles' continuous demand for oxygen. Examples of aerobic exercise include brisk walking, dancing, step aerobics, running or jogging, and biking.

Alzheimer's disease: A progressive, incurable condition that destroys brain cells, gradually causing loss of intellectual abilities such as memory and extreme changes in personality and behavior.

amenorrhea: Absence or cessation of menstrual periods.

androgens: Male sex hormones, such as *testosterone*, that are produced by the *adrenal glands* in both males and females. The *ovaries* secrete very small amounts of androgens until *menopause*.

anemia: A blood disorder caused by a deficiency of red blood cells or hemoglobin (the oxygen-carrying protein in red blood cells), which can result from heavy menstrual bleeding.

angina: A tight, heavy, squeezing sensation deep beneath the breastbone or in a band across the chest that results from a reduced supply of oxygen to the heart muscle, indicating heart disease. The pain may also radiate to the left arm, shoulder, neck, jaw, or down the back and be accompanied by nausea, sweating, or shortness of breath.

anorexia nervosa: A potentially life-threatening eating disorder (most frequent in young women) characterized by an abnormal fear of becoming fat, prolonged avoidance of food, and excessive weight loss.

anovulation: Failure of the ovaries to produce, nurture, or release mature eggs.

antigen: A foreign substance capable of stimulating an immune response in the body. The immune system reacts by producing antibodies to fight the antigen.

antioxidants: Compounds that protect against cell damage inflicted by molecules called oxygen *free radicals*, which are a major cause of disease and aging.

artery: One of the large blood vessels that carries oxygen-filled blood away from your heart to your organs and tissues.

atheroma: Fatty deposits on the inner lining of an *artery* that can lead to *atherosclerosis*.

atherosclerosis: The buildup of fatty material called *plaque* in the inner lining of arteries, which can narrow the blood vessels and reduce blood flow through them.

autologous blood donation: Donation of a person's own blood before scheduled elective surgery to make the blood available in case a transfusion is necessary during or after surgery.

B

benign: Describes an abnormal growth that is noncancerous.

biopsy: A diagnostic test in which small samples of tissue are removed from the body and examined under a microscope.

bladder: A hollow, muscular organ in the *pelvis* that acts as a reservoir for urine.

blood pressure: A measure of the force exerted against the walls of arteries by the flow of blood as it is pumped by the heart to the rest of the body.

bone density: A measure of the amount of calcium and other minerals in bone in relation to the width of the bone; used to determine the risk of developing *osteoporosis*.

C

CA-125 test: A blood test to detect an elevated level of an *antigen* called CA-125, which may indicate ovarian cancer; however, the test is not exact, so further testing must be done to make a definitive diagnosis.

calcium: A mineral that gives strength to bones and teeth and also has an important role in muscle contraction, blood clotting, and nerve function.

carcinogen: Any agent, such as cigarette smoke, that is capable of causing cancer.

carcinoma in situ: An abnormal growth in the surface layer or lining of a body structure with cells that show *precancerous* changes but no tendency to invade other tissues.

cardiovascular system: The network formed by your heart and blood vessels that pumps blood and carries it throughout your body; also called **circulatory system**.

catheter: A hollow, flexible tube that is inserted into a vessel or body cavity to withdraw or instill fluids or to widen a passageway.

cervical dysplasia: A condition in which cells in the *cervix* have undergone *precancerous* changes that can be detected by a *Pap smear*; treatment can prevent it from becoming cancerous.

cervix: The neck and lower part of the *uterus* that separates the cavity of the uterus from the vagina.

chemotherapy: Treatment of cancer using powerful drugs to destroy cancer cells throughout the body.

cholesterol: A fatlike substance that is an important constituent of cells and is involved in the transport of fats in the blood; a high level of it in the blood increases the risk of heart disease.

colposcopy: Visual examination of the *cervix* and *vagina* using a lighted magnifying instrument (colposcope) inserted through the vagina.

cone biopsy: Surgical removal of a cone-shaped section of tissue from the *cervix* for examination under a microscope.

cyst: An abnormal lump or swelling filled with fluid or semisolid material.

cystitis: Inflammation of the inner lining of the *bladder*, usually caused by a bacterial infection.

cystocele: A condition in which weakened pelvic muscles cause the base of the *bladder* to drop from its usual position down into the *vagina*.

D

D & C (dilation and curettage): A surgical procedure in which the *cervix* is dilated (widened) and the lining of the *uterus* is scraped away; used to diagnose and treat disorders of the uterus, such as heavy vaginal bleeding.

DEXA (dual energy X-ray absorptiometry): The most effective imaging technique used to measure *bone density*. DEXA uses a very low dose of radiation and can detect bone loss of as little as 1 percent. The procedure is painless and takes from 3 to 7 minutes.

diabetes: A disorder in which the body is unable to properly use the sugar *glucose*; its two forms are type I (insulin-dependent) diabetes and type II (non–insulin-dependent) diabetes.

diastolic blood pressure: The second, lower number in a *blood pressure* reading indicating the pressure in the vessels when the heart rests between beats and fills with blood.

DPA (dual photon absorptiometry): An imaging technique that measures *bone density* in the spine, neck, and hips using a very low dose of radiation. DPA is used to determine the need for *HRT* in postmenopausal women who have broken a bone. The procedure is painless and takes from 20 to 40 minutes.

dysmenorrhea: Pain or discomfort experienced just before or during a menstrual period.

E

embolism: Interruption of blood flow in a blood vessel obstructed by an *embolus.*

embolus: A plug of material (such as a blood clot or an air bubble) that can travel in the bloodstream and block a blood vessel.

endometrial hyperplasia: Abnormal thickening of the *endometrium* caused by excessive cell growth.

endometriosis: A condition in which tissue resembling that of the *endometrium* grows outside the *uterus*, on or near the *ovaries* or *fallopian tubes*, or in other areas of the abdominal cavity.

endometrium: The inner lining of the wall of the *uterus* that thickens during each menstrual cycle and is shed in menstrual blood.

endorphins: Chemicals produced in the brain that can improve mood and help control response to pain and stress.

endoscopy: A procedure that uses a lighted viewing instrument (endoscope) to look inside a body cavity or organ to diagnose or treat disorders.

enterocele: A condition caused by weakened muscles in the pelvis in which a portion of the intestines bulges into the top of the vagina, sometimes causing recurring pain in the lower back.

estrogen: The key female hormone, produced mostly in the ovaries, that carries messages to many types of cells; it is essential for the healthy development and functioning of the female reproductive system and also plays a critical role in keeping bones strong and brain cells healthy. See *HRT* regarding estrogen medications.

F

fallopian tubes: Two thin tubes that extend from either side of the *uterus* to an *ovary*, where they flare out and are open to receive an egg during each menstrual cycle; each tube is a passageway for eggs and sperm and the site of fertilization.

fibroids: Noncancerous growths in or on the *uterus* that develop from muscle cells in the wall of the uterus.

folic acid: An essential B vitamin during early pregnancy that helps prevent birth defects in the fetus.

free radicals: Molecules produced in the body (by normal cell activity or by external agents such as radiation and cigarette smoke) that damage cells; they play a major role in disease and aging.

FSH (follicle-stimulating hormone): A hormone secreted by the *pituitary gland* that stimulates the growth and maturation of eggs in females and sperm in males.

G

glucose: A simple sugar that is the main source of energy for cells.

gonadotropin-releasing hormone (GnRH): A hormone secreted by the *hypothalamus*, which stimulates the *pituitary gland* to produce *FSH* and *LH*, the gonadotropic hormones.

H

HDL (high density lipoprotein): A type of fat carried in the blood-stream, often referred to as the "good" *cholesterol*, that protects against heart disease by cleansing blood vessels of the "bad" cholesterol (*LDL*).

heartbeat: A contraction of the heart muscle that pumps blood into the *arteries* and throughout the body.

heart rate: The number of *heartbeats* per minute.

hemoglobin: The oxygen-carrying protein in red blood cells.

hormone replacement therapy: See *HRT*.

hormones: Chemicals, such as *estrogen* and *progesterone*, that are produced by the body and released directly into the bloodstream to perform specific functions.

hot flash: A sudden wave of heat that typically starts in the upper chest and neck and spreads upward to the face and down the shoulders. A hot flash may last from a few seconds to a few minutes or longer and is often followed by flushing, perspiration, and a cold, clammy feeling as the body temperature readjusts. Hot flashes are usually associated with decreased *estrogen* production at *menopause*.

HRT (hormone replacement therapy): The use of hormones, such as the female hormones *estrogen* and *progestin*, as medication to replace those hormones the body no longer produces naturally.

hydrogenated fats: Vegetable oils that have been converted into a solid form, such as stick margarine or canned shortening; these fats can raise the level of harmful *LDL* cholesterol in the blood.

hyperplasia, endometrial: Excessive growth of cells in the *endometrium*.

hypertension: A condition in which *blood pressure* is persistently raised; a major risk factor for *stroke*.

hypothalamus: A small structure at the base of the brain that regulates many body functions, including appetite and body temperature.

hysterectomy: Surgical removal of the *uterus*.

hysterosalpingography: X-ray examination of the *uterus* and *fallopian tubes* to investigate the cause of infertility.

hysteroscopy: Visual examination of the *cervix* and the interior of the *uterus* using a viewing instrument (hysteroscope) inserted through the vagina.

I

incontinence, urinary: Uncontrollable, involuntary leaking of urine.

inhibin: A substance secreted by the *ovaries* that inhibits the production of *FSH* by the *pituitary gland*.

ischemia: Temporary decrease in the supply of oxygen to an organ or tissue.

K

Kegel exercises: Exercises that strengthen the muscles of the pelvic floor. Kegel exercises are used to treat pelvic support problems such as *urinary incontinence*.

kidneys: The two abdominal organs that filter waste products and excess water from the blood. The kidneys play an essential role in maintaining *blood pressure*.

L

laparoscopy: Examination of or surgery in the abdomen using a viewing tube (laparoscope) and instruments inserted through tiny incisions in the abdomen.

LDL (low density lipoprotein): A type of fat carried in the bloodstream that is often referred to as the "bad" *cholesterol* because it increases the risk of *atherosclerosis* and heart disease.

LH (luteinizing hormone): A hormone secreted by the *pituitary gland* that stimulates the growth and maturation of eggs in females and sperm in males.

libido: Sexual desire; loss of libido can be a symptom of *menopause*.

lymph nodes: Small glands clustered in the neck, armpits, abdomen, and groin that supply infection-fighting cells to the bloodstream and filter out bacteria and other *antigens*.

M

malignant: Describes a condition, such as cancer, that tends to become progressively worse and can be fatal.

mammography: An X-ray procedure for detecting breast cancer at an early, curable stage.

menopause: The cessation of a woman's menstrual periods, usually sometime between ages 40 and 55; also refers to the years leading up to the final period.

metastasis: The spread of cancer from its original site in the body.

myocardial infarction (MI): Sudden death of a section of the heart muscle because of a loss of blood supply. The most common cause of MI is blockage of blood flow in one of the coronary *arteries* by a *thrombus* (blood clot). Symptoms include severe, constant chest pain; shortness of breath; nausea; vomiting; restlessness; cold, clammy skin; and loss of consciousness. Risk factors for MI include stress, high blood levels of *cholesterol*, *atherosclerosis*, *obesity*, *diabetes mellitus*, and *hypertension*. Also called **heart attack.**

myomectomy: A surgical procedure to remove *fibroids* from the *uterus*, leaving the uterus intact.

O

obesity: A condition in which a person weighs 20 percent or more over the maximum desirable weight for his or her build and height.

oophorectomy: Surgical removal of one or both *ovaries.*

osteoarthritis: Progressive, gradual thinning or destruction of cartilage in the joints, usually resulting from injury or overuse.

osteoporosis: A disorder in which bones thin and become brittle and more prone to fracture; most common in women after *menopause.*

ovaries: A pair of glands located on either side of the *uterus,* directly below the *fallopian tubes.* The ovaries produce eggs and the female sex hormones, *estrogen* and *progesterone.*

ovulation: The cyclic release of an egg from an *ovary.*

P

Pap smear: A test in which cells are scraped from the surface of the *cervix* and examined under a microscope to detect abnormal cells that are or could become cancerous.

parathyroid glands: Two pairs of glands located in the neck, near the thyroid gland. The parathyroid glands produce parathyroid hormone, which helps control the level of *calcium* in the blood.

pelvis: The basin-shaped bony structure at the base of the spine, consisting of the ilium (hipbone), the sacrum, and the coccyx. The pelvis protects abdominal organs, such as the *bladder, ovaries,* and *uterus.*

perimenopause: The transitional period that leads up to *menopause.* Women in perimenopause may experience changes in their menstrual cycle and may also have *hot flashes.*

pessary: A rubber device that is inserted through the vagina to help hold the *uterus* in place in women who have *prolapse of the uterus*.

pituitary gland: A gland at the base of the brain that secretes hormones and regulates and controls other hormone-secreting glands and many body processes, including reproduction.

plaque, arterial: Fatty material that builds up inside artery walls; this buildup can eventually narrow or block the blood vessel, causing a heart attack or stroke.

PMS (premenstrual syndrome): A range of physical and emotional symptoms that some women experience in the 7 to 10 days preceding their period.

polyp: A growth that projects, usually on a stalk, from a membrane in the body and can sometimes develop into cancer.

potassium: An essential mineral needed by your body to maintain water balance, conduct nerve signals, contract muscles, and sustain a normal heart rhythm.

precancerous: Describes any condition that has a potential to become cancerous.

progesterone: A female sex hormone produced by the *ovaries* that is essential for a healthy pregnancy.

progestin: A synthetic form of *progesterone* often taken in *HRT*.

prolapse of the uterus: Displacement of the *uterus* down into the vagina caused by a weakening of supporting tissues in the pelvis.

psychotherapy: Describes a variety of treatments for mental or emotional disorders that are used to help people change their behavior and experience through techniques such as talking, reinforcement, reassurance, and support.

pulse: Rhythmic expansion and contraction of an *artery* as blood is pumped through it.

R

radiation therapy: Treatment, usually for cancer, using X rays or other forms of radiation to destroy or slow the spread of cancer cells.

rectocele: A condition in which weakening of the vaginal wall causes the rectum to bulge into the vagina.

S

salpingectomy: Surgical removal of one or both *fallopian tubes.*

salt sensitive: A term used to describe a person whose *blood pressure* goes up and down in relation to the amount of salt (*sodium*) in his or her diet.

saturated fat: A type of fat in the diet, found in meats and dairy products, that can raise the level of *cholesterol* in the blood and increase the risk of heart disease and some cancers.

sodium: An essential mineral that helps your body maintain water balance and *blood pressure.* Your body also needs sodium to conduct nerve signals and contract muscles. Too much salt in the diet may contribute to *hypertension* in people who are *salt sensitive.* Sodium is found in table salt.

stress incontinence: Involuntary leaking of urine during activities that increase pressure inside the abdomen, such as coughing, sneezing, or jogging.

stroke: Damage to part of the brain caused by an interruption in blood flow to the area. Ischemic stroke, the most common type, results from blockage of a blood vessel in the brain. Hemorrhagic stroke results from a ruptured blood vessel in the brain.

systolic blood pressure: The first, higher number in a *blood pressure* reading indicating the pressure in the vessels when the heart beats and pumps blood into the circulation.

T

testosterone: The key male sex hormone that stimulates bone and muscle growth and the development of male sex characteristics.

thrombosis, deep vein: Formation of blood clots in veins deep inside the legs, usually resulting from sluggish blood flow caused by lack of activity.

thrombus: A blood clot (a clump of coagulated blood) that forms inside a blood vessel. When a blood clot breaks off and travels through the bloodstream, it is called an *embolus*.

thyroid gland: A gland located in your neck that secretes *hormones* that are essential for regulating various processes that occur in your body, including your *heart rate* and *blood pressure*.

transient ischemic attack (TIA): A brief interruption in blood flow to the brain, causing temporary symptoms such as impaired vision, sensation, movement, or speech.

triglycerides: The major fats in the blood; a high level indicates an increased risk of heart disease, *hypertension*, and *diabetes*.

U

ultrasound: A diagnostic imaging procedure that uses high-frequency sound waves to create a picture of internal body structures on a video screen.

unsaturated fat: A type of fat found in most vegetable oils that does not raise *cholesterol* levels in the blood.

ureters: The two tubes that carry urine from the *kidneys* to the *bladder*.

urethra: The narrow channel through which urine passes from the *bladder* out of the body.

urinary incontinence: See *incontinence, urinary*.

uterus: The hollow, muscular organ in the center of the female pelvis that sheds its lining each month during menstruation and in which a fertilized egg implants and grows into a fetus.

V

vagina: The muscular passageway that connects the *cervix* with the *vulva*.

vaginal hysterectomy: An operation in which the *uterus* is removed through the *vagina*. Vaginal hysterectomy produces less pain and requires a slightly shorter hospitalization and recovery time than does abdominal hysterectomy.

vaginal ultrasound: An *ultrasound* procedure in which a thin wand inserted into the *vagina* emits sound waves that produce an image of the *ovaries* and other reproductive organs.

vein: A blood vessel that returns blood from your organs and tissues to your heart.

vulva: The external, visible part of the female genitalia.

Index

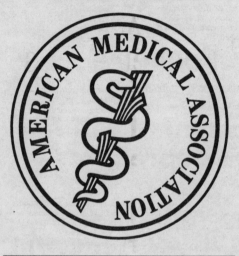
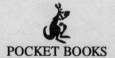

ALSO FROM THE
American Medical Association
AND
Pocket Books:

Essential Guide to Depression

•

Essential Guide to Hypertension

•

Essential Guide to Asthma

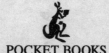

POCKET BOOKS